20 +
TRUE STORIES
OF DISABILITY AND
DETERMINATION

DOWN SYNDROME OUT LOUD

BY MELISSA HART   ILLUSTRATED BY MARÍA PERERA

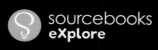

sourcebooks
eXplore

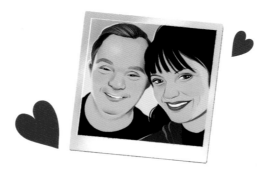

For my brother Mark, the inspiration for this book, and for our
mother—a tireless champion for full inclusion of all people.

Text © 2025 by Melissa Hart
Illustrations © 2025 by María Perera
Cover and internal design © 2025 by Sourcebooks
Cover design by Maryn Arreguín / Sourcebooks
Internal design by Jessica Nordskog / Sourcebooks

Published by eXplore, an imprint of Sourcebooks Kids
P.O. Box 4410, Naperville, Illinois 60567-4410
(630) 961-3900
sourcebooks.com

Cataloging-in-Publication Data is on file with the Library of Congress.

Source of Production: Leo Paper, Heshan City, Guangdong Province, China
Date of Production: December 2024
Run Number: 5042353

Printed and bound in China.
LEO 10 9 8 7 6 5 4 3 2 1

TABLE OF CONTENTS

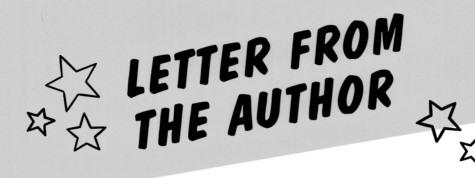

LETTER FROM THE AUTHOR

DEAR READERS,

When I was five years old, my little brother was born. His name was Mark, and he was an adorable baby with fine blond hair and chubby cheeks. My mother told me that he had Down syndrome. I didn't know what that was. I only knew that I loved Mark, and we played together all the time.

Flash-forward to middle school, where I was a shy, quiet bookworm who loved music and nature. I would sit on the floor of Mark's bedroom and play the guitar while we sang our favorite songs, like "Puff the Magic Dragon" and "Memory" from the Broadway musical *Cats*. Mark couldn't walk that far on his little seven-year-old legs because of his poor muscle tone—common in kids with Down syndrome—so I pulled him in a yellow wagon to our local park. We played on the merry-go-round, the swings, and the slide, and we had picnics under the oak trees. Sometimes we would argue, but I never felt embarrassed about Mark in front of others. Mark was one of my best friends when we were kids.

As Mark and I grew older, I noticed that sometimes people treated him unkindly. They stared at him and pointed. One time, he said hello to a little girl in a grocery store, and her mother yanked her away, saying, "Don't talk to people like him!" Another time, a kid at the Boys and Girls Club called him the r-word. In response, my brother karate kicked him. (I put that scene in my novel *Avenging the Owl*.) And then there was the night we went to a Halloween party in my university town, and college boys made fun of Mark...until Michael Jackson's "Thriller" came on and Mark grabbed everyone's attention with his incredible dance moves. I beamed, proud that he was my brother.

These days, Mark and I live in separate states, but we talk on the phone every night. Mark loves to bowl and run track with his Special Olympics team. He's a huge sports fan, so he watches baseball, basketball, or football every night. He listens to country music and works as a dishwasher at Texas Roadhouse. He has a great sense of humor, always making me laugh with his impersonation of the Three Stooges and his dad jokes.

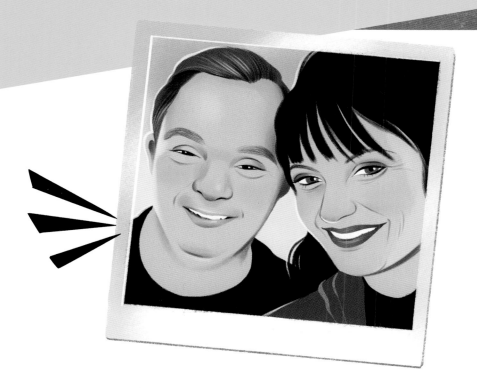

I wrote *Down Syndrome Out Loud* because I wanted to learn more about people with the genetic condition my brother has. In my research and interviews, I learned that people with Down syndrome do amazing things. They're U.S. Congressional lobbyists committed to advocating for the rights of people with disabilities. They're actors and comedians breaking barriers on stage and screen. They're athletes and dancers and teachers and entrepreneurs, inspiring people with their talents. Like Mark, they value family and close friendships. They work toward goals, and they have good days and bad days. They respond to discrimination with frustration and anger, and they fight to be included in all aspects of life.

I hope my book inspires you to befriend the people around you who have Down syndrome and other disabilities. I hope you'll include them on your sports teams, in your clubs, at your birthday parties, and in everyday life. Inclusion shows us that we're not that different from one another. We learn that other kids don't have to look like us or even sound like us to be great friends. Inclusion widens our circles of friendship and teaches us that everyone has so much to contribute to this world. My own life is much richer—and much more interesting— because of my friendship with my brother and other people with disabilities. Yours will be as well.

AMAZING PEOPLE

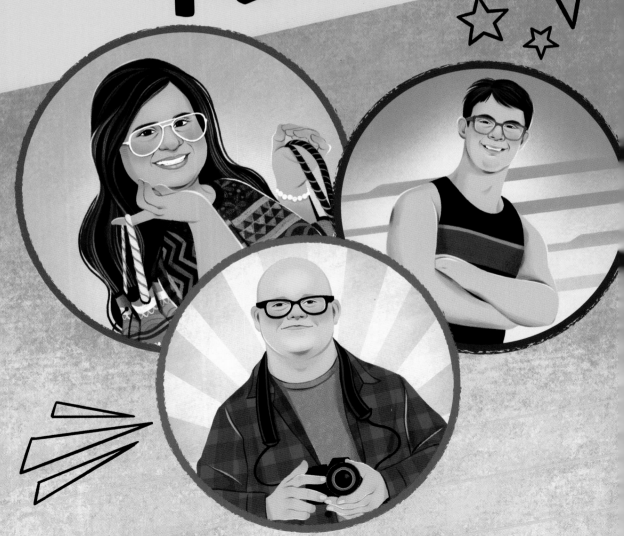

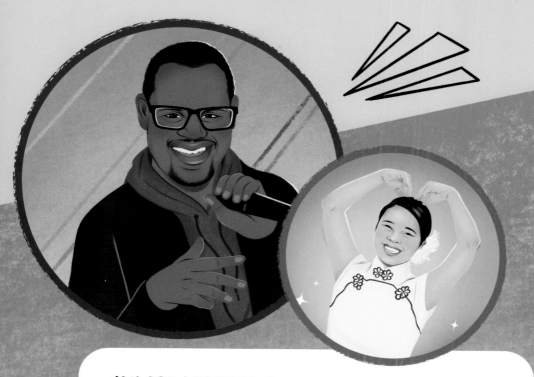

YOU ARE ABOUT TO MEET some amazing people! They were all born with a genetic condition called Down syndrome. Learning to walk and talk and read and write proved more challenging for them than for most kids born without this condition. Some suffered bullying in school because they looked and sounded a little different than their classmates. Some dealt with discrimination when they applied for college or a job. Many worked for years and years with physical therapists, speech therapists, and doctors. But all of them—with the help of family and friends—overcame these challenges to fulfill their dreams. You'll meet actors and athletes, teachers and artists, entrepreneurs and activists—each with their own story of how they worked to achieve personal goals. Today, they strive to ensure the basic rights of a group of people who used to be hidden away and silenced. This is Down syndrome out loud!

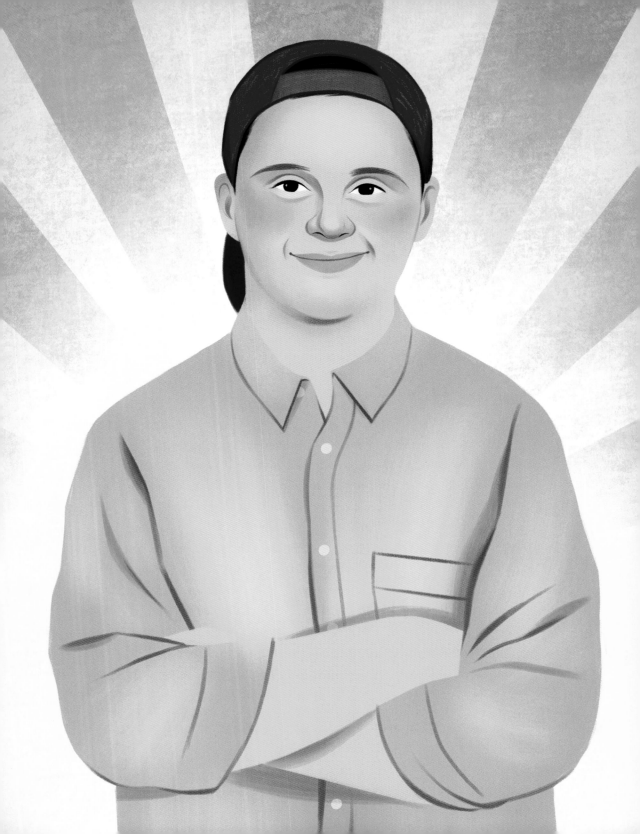

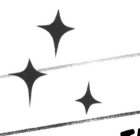

ALEX BOURNE:
THE WORLD TRAVELER

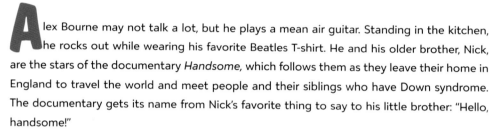

Home Country: England • Born in 1995

Alex Bourne may not talk a lot, but he plays a mean air guitar. Standing in the kitchen, he rocks out while wearing his favorite Beatles T-shirt. He and his older brother, Nick, are the stars of the documentary *Handsome,* which follows them as they leave their home in England to travel the world and meet people and their siblings who have Down syndrome. The documentary gets its name from Nick's favorite thing to say to his little brother: "Hello, handsome!"

Things weren't always as wonderful as they are now for Alex and Nick. When he was younger, Nick felt a bit ashamed of Alex. Nick wanted to fit in with the rest of his teenage friends, and he didn't want to include his younger brother with Down syndrome.

Alex was a naturally happy person, but he was also soft-spoken and shy, and he had difficulty communicating in words. When teachers found that he couldn't keep up with his peers in his mainstream school, they sent him out of the classroom to watch TV. So he and his family moved to Hampshire, where Alex attended special education classes at a school that offered students the opportunity to work on a farm and practice living skills in a residential house.

Later, Alex watched Nick go off to drama school in London. In that school, teachers asked students to visualize someone they'd fight for, and Nick kept picturing Alex. Older and wiser, he realized his brother was awesome, and he wanted to spend more time with him. When Nick returned home, he found that he loved to joke, laugh, and wrestle with Alex. Nick even invited Alex to move in with him!

Nick couldn't find any movies or books about people with Down syndrome and their siblings. He wanted to create a resource to help other teens better understand their siblings with the condition. He thought of writing a book, but their mother suggested he make a documentary instead. Since Nick was a professionally trained actor, this made so much sense!

Nick and Alex decided to make a documentary they'd call *Handsome*. First, they asked two filmmakers, Nick's friends Ed and Luke, to move in with them and film whatever they wanted. It took a little time, but Alex got used to having Ed and Luke around, and he learned to go about living his daily life. The filmmakers caught him on video doing two of his favorite things—dancing and singing at the top of his lungs.

One time, Ed and Luke followed the brothers on a road trip to Cornwall in their rented vintage VW bus. Alex played football and went to the pub with Charlie, another young man with Down syndrome. They chatted with Charlie's mother, who described how doctors had advised her to send him away so he wouldn't ruin his siblings' lives. (She ignored them!) Alex's project with Nick proved so illuminating that they raised money to travel around the world to meet other people with Down syndrome and their brothers and sisters.

One of the most exciting places they visited was India. The shy, quiet kid that Alex used to be when he struggled in class learned to cross hot, busy streets in Mumbai and play cricket on the beach! He danced to traditional Indian music with his new friend Sagit, who also has Down syndrome. Alex and Nick found that they had so much in common with Sagit and his brother Krish despite living thousands of miles apart.

Ed and Luke also filmed Alex and Nick traveling to New York City and to Vietnam, where they discovered different perspectives about people with disabilities. Alex observed firsthand that some adults in Vietnam put people with Down syndrome in institutions, far away from their families. Fortunately, Alex remembers the good parts of that trip most vividly—in particular the delicious chicken and noodles he enjoyed on the street.

Handsome premiered at the 2021 Glasgow Film Festival in Scotland. The film review website Movie Marker called it "a heart-swelling and eye-opening exploration of an everyday life misunderstood by many." It's since gone to streaming services where everyone in the world can watch it.

These days, Alex lives with his mother and father southwest of London. He gets up early, excited to see what the new day holds for him. He's an excellent bowler, and he plays miniature golf, football, and basketball. Alex is learning photography and woodwork; he's a devoted sports fan and loves films that make him laugh out loud—like *Mrs. Doubtfire*—and humorous TV shows including the 1960s–70s British sitcom *Dad's Army*.

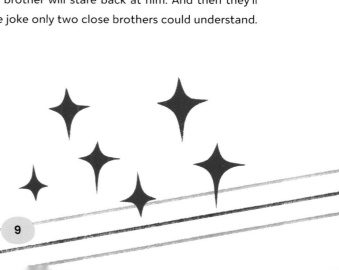

Alex's favorite band is the Beatles—especially the album *Let It Be*—and the singer John Lennon. He likes to listen to music, go to country music concerts in London, and walk his friends' dogs. For fun, Alex goes to the local pub with his family and friends and orders lemonade and cheese and onion crisps (called chips in the U.S.); they might also play a game of snooker, which is a bit like billiards in the U.S.

Alex loves to go on a journey. He particularly enjoys the coast of Cornwall, where he wades in the ocean and orders Mars ice cream bars. In the summer of 2023, he traveled to France with his older brother and sister-in-law, where he adored taking photos of the beautiful mountains. He's lately become Uncle Alex to Nick's daughter and loves to spend time with their family. Every so often, he'll look at Nick—just as he did by the campfire during the filming of *Handsome*—and his brother will stare back at him. And then they'll both burst out laughing...sharing an inside joke only two close brothers could understand.

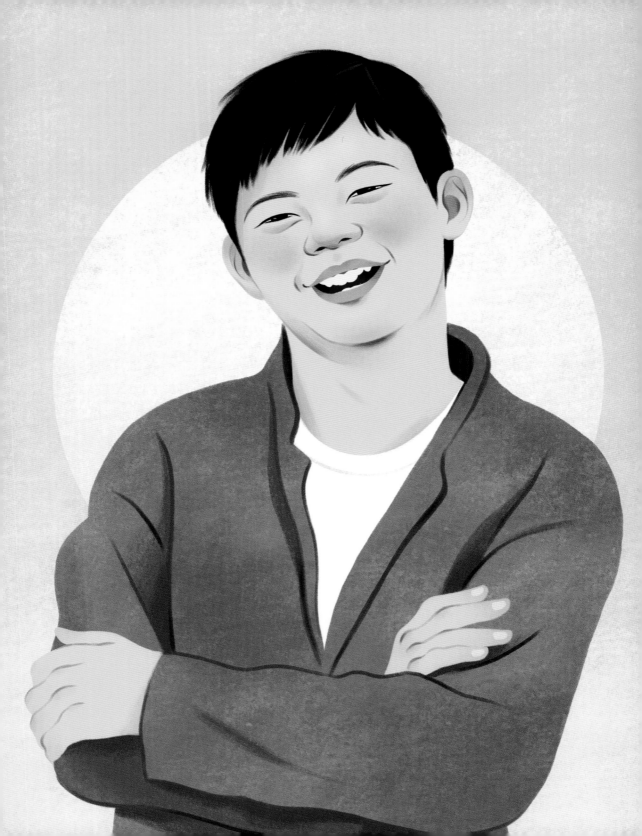

ALEX LEE: THE SELF-ADVOCATE

Home Country: The United States • Born in 2007

Alex Lee was a seventh grader when he, his mother, and his older sister, Isabelle, strolled in the rain past the rows of colorful flags into the United Nations building in New York City. Alex had been invited to give the closing remarks at the World Down Syndrome Day Conference that year, an event attended by hundreds of people.

In a crisp white shirt and suit and tie, he sat at the front of the room in the vast chambers and spoke into the microphone. "Many people think people with Down syndrome have a lot of limitations, but I think that's so wrong," he said. "I speak, read, and write in two languages, English and Korean. I sing opera in Italian and do public speaking."

Alex Lee has been a public speaker and a passionate advocate for inclusive education since he was eight years old. He grew up in Pennsylvania, fully included in school classrooms starting in preschool. His parents emigrated to the U.S. from Korea before he and Isabelle were born. Though some doctors said that teaching Alex two languages at once would confuse him, his family members ignored their advice. He became one of the first children in his classroom to read, and his best friend, Charlie, begged him to read stories out loud.

Alex originally believed the people who said math was difficult for those with Down syndrome. He struggled with math and had difficulty adding and subtracting in his head... until a teacher gave him a calculator. Suddenly, a whole world opened up to him. Alex memorized formulas, learned to calculate the volume of various shapes, and regularly earned As on his math tests.

In school, Alex has always worked with a paraeducator, a teacher who sits with him in classes and helps him with the more challenging assignments. "It makes a huge difference to be able to lean on my para, Mr. G.," Alex explains of his high school support staff. "He knows what I can do and when I need a little more help. Plus, because I've been included since preschool, everyone knows me, and I know that they always have my back. When I'm struggling, there's always a friend or two I can buddy up with to try and work through something. I'm really happy about that."

Sometimes, Mr. G. and Alex even get a bit mischievous. Typically, they use the study hall period to catch up on whatever work Alex hasn't done for the day. But several times, Alex sent Mr. G. out for his favorite strawberry ice cream, promising to work independently. Then they'd pretend they needed to work on a project in an empty room. "But really," Alex says, "we'd sit and eat ice cream."

As a fourth grader, Alex visited his senator's office in Washington, DC, to explain how inclusion in regular classrooms had benefited him. "I learn with all my friends, everything from sedimentary rocks to the state bird of Ohio," he said at a large table full of kids with disabilities and their parents. "I really like science and social studies, but I have to say that recess is my favorite part of school, just like all of the other fourth graders."

In fifth grade, Alex visited the United Nations for the first time, delivering remarks for World Down Syndrome Day. "I believe getting an education and being able to feel a sense of growing in school and in the community is a basic right for every person, including people with Down syndrome."

That same summer, Alex talked to hundreds of teachers at the Office of Special Education Programs Leadership Conference about inclusion.

In middle school, Alex became a member of the National Junior Honor Society and joined his school's chapter of Best Buddies, an organization that matches people with disabilities with nondisabled peers as friends (see page 112). Alex's love of math followed him to middle and high school. "I like spending time on problems and really making an effort to crack them," he says. "It's like a puzzle. I'm really passionate about it." And although his high school English teacher worried that he might not be able to keep up with the required reading for the class, Alex proved adept at reading *Romeo and Juliet*. He even played Friar Laurence in a classroom production of Shakespeare's play. He joined the high school multicultural music club too. "I love listening to music in my free time," he says.

When he's not at school, Alex loves to play *Mario Kart* with his friends. "I like chilling and talking," he adds. He also loves to cook with his sister. Together, they've perfected their recipes for seafood pasta and garlic bread. Alex loves to watch soccer on TV, particularly the Tottenham Hotspurs from England. His favorite films are *The Boss Baby* and *Pee-wee's Big Adventure*. "Alex and Pee-wee have the same sense of humor," his mother says.

Alex hopes to attend Swarthmore College, where his sister is attending, where he'll major in math and continue advocating for the educational rights of kids with disabilities. The Departments of Education of several states have invited him to speak to their teachers and staff.

"I like to share my story and let people know how awesome inclusion really is and how much it changes life for kids like me," Alex says. "Whenever I speak, I think the most important thing is that I've inspired someone to believe in inclusion and to want to change things for the better for people with Down syndrome."

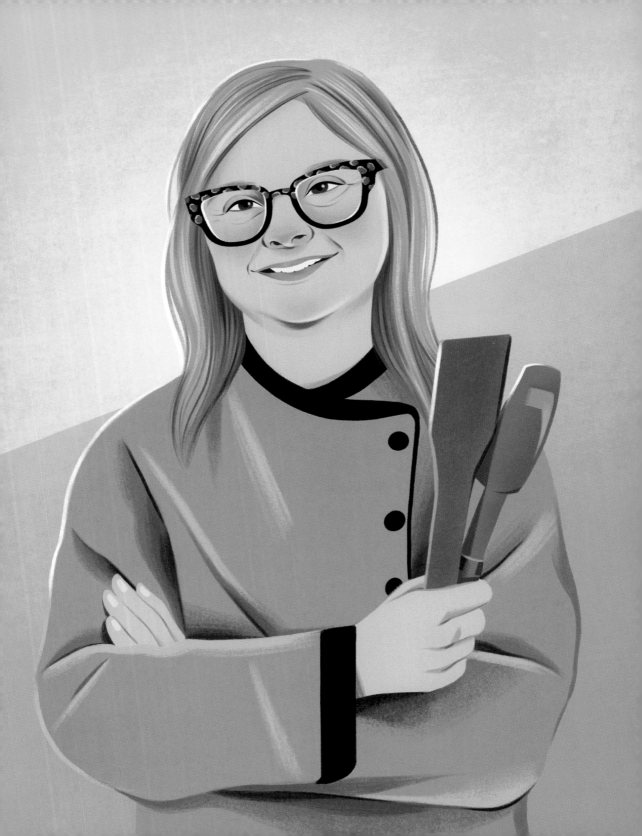

ALLISON FOGARTY: THE DOG TREAT BAKER

Home Country: The United States • Born in 1991

Allison Fogarty bends over an oven in her lime-green chef's jacket with her sparkly manicure protected by heat-resistant gloves. With Lady Gaga playing in the background, she pulls out a tray of homemade dog treats shaped like tiny bones. She places the tray on a rack to cool, and her pink smartwatch buzzes. It's another order for Doggy Delights by Allison, her business specializing in all-natural dog treats shipped all over the U.S.

"Cooking is my passion," she says. "I love to cook for people, but cooking for dogs is something I can do by myself."

Allison was born and raised in Chicago, Illinois. In addition to being born with Down syndrome, she had a tracheoesophageal fistula and laryngeal cleft. Allison had so many health issues that doctors had to insert a trach tube in her neck to help her breathe when she was an infant. Still, she attended elementary school with her typical peers. She adored the school nurse who, concerned about how little Allison weighed, brought her french fries from McDonald's. "I loved to eat french fries all the time when I was little," Allison says.

At one point, when she was eleven, Allison's health conditions deteriorated. Luckily, her ENT located her previously undiscovered laryngeal cleft. The doctors told her she had to have multiple surgeries; most importantly, a G-tube would be inserted into her stomach to protect her airway. Throughout middle school, she wasn't allowed to eat or drink by mouth.

That was a rough time for Allison. She spent weeks at a time in the hospital and coped by watching cooking shows on the Food Network. She especially loved watching celebrity chef Rachael Ray. "She saved my life," Allison says. "She made delicious food, and that made me feel like I wanted to be a chef like her. I wished I didn't have a G-tube, so I could eat and drink again and be a chef."

Eventually Allison got well enough to attend high school and participate in Special Olympics and Best Buddies. She also acted in a local theater troupe and played many roles, including Miss Hannigan in a production of *Annie*. Another favorite role was Prudy Singleton in the musical *Hairspray*, which is about a teenager who battles racism while trying to land a role as a dancer on a local TV show.

"You gotta think big to be big," she says, quoting her favorite line. Like Tracy in *Hairspray*, Allison was a nonconformist. "I did not follow directions, and I got in trouble a lot," she admits of her time in school.

After she graduated, various agencies supporting people with disabilities told her she wouldn't be able to find a job because of her poor health, so she and her mother, Pat, started a business called Lunch Break. For three years, Allison cooked and delivered thirty lunches a week to Pat's former coworkers at a local school. Then, in 2017, Allison's parents decided to move from Illinois to Florida.

"At first, I didn't like it at all," Allison admits. "I didn't want to leave my family and friends. The move broke my heart."

Fortunately, the Down Syndrome Association of Central Florida had just launched an Entrepreneur Academy for adults with Down syndrome who were eager to start businesses. At first, Allison and her mother tried to make cat treats, but their four cats wouldn't eat them. Because she'd met so many dogs in her new neighborhood, she decided to try a dog business instead. Allison immediately began testing recipes for dog treats and came up with Yogurt and Berry Delights, Salmon Training Treats, and Peanut Butter Delights, which her niece liked to sample. For two years, Allison sold her treats at the local farmers market, where she became friends with many of the local dogs. Her favorite was a dog named Moose. She nicknamed him Chocolate Mousse.

In 2018, Allison's mom wrote to Rachael Ray who, a whole year later, invited Allison to appear on her show via FaceTime. During that show (January 2019), Rachael invited Allison to make dog treats with her in New York. In the three-minute clip that aired in August 2020, Rachael and Allison made sweet potato dog treats together, and Rachael even sampled one. "These are delicious, by the way," Rachael said. "You can even share them with your dog!"

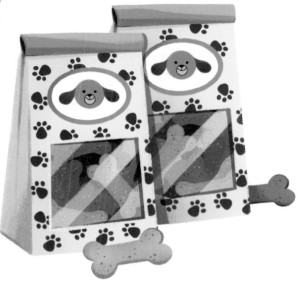

After Allison appeared on *The Rachael Ray Show*, orders for Doggy Delights by Allison exploded. She and her family purchased three freeze dryers, which Allison nicknamed Eenie, Meeny, and Moe. Allison bakes and packages her dog treats, including a personal letter every time that reads "I hope you enjoy your delicious and healthy biscuits, homemade with LOVE by me—Allison."

These days, Allison puts on her lime-green chef's coat and gets to work in the spacious kitchen she shares with her parents. She loves to make an assembly line of ingredients (the way Rachael Ray does on her cooking shows) before mixing up the dog treat batter. "It takes forever to put them in the molds and bake them," she says. "That part isn't my favorite. But I love dogs, and I want to pet them. It's so fun to see when they love my treats."

In her free time, Allison goes to Friendship Club. "It's for people with Down syndrome and disabilities, and we do different activities," she says. She also likes to play card games like Hand and Foot at the neighborhood clubhouse and Bunco with her mother and their friends. Allison loves to watch horror movies like *Boogeyman 2 and Insidious* with her boyfriend, Brent, and then go out to dinner.

Aside from being a dog treat chef, Allison works as a motivational speaker all over Florida. Her main presentation is "Entrepreneurship: Your Dreams Can Come True." In a speech for the Annual Family Café—a motivational conference for people with disabilities—she stood at the podium in her lime-green chef's jacket and smiled. "This is the perfect job for me," she told an audience made up of people with Down syndrome and their families. "Every day, I wake up and think about my job and what I will cook that day."

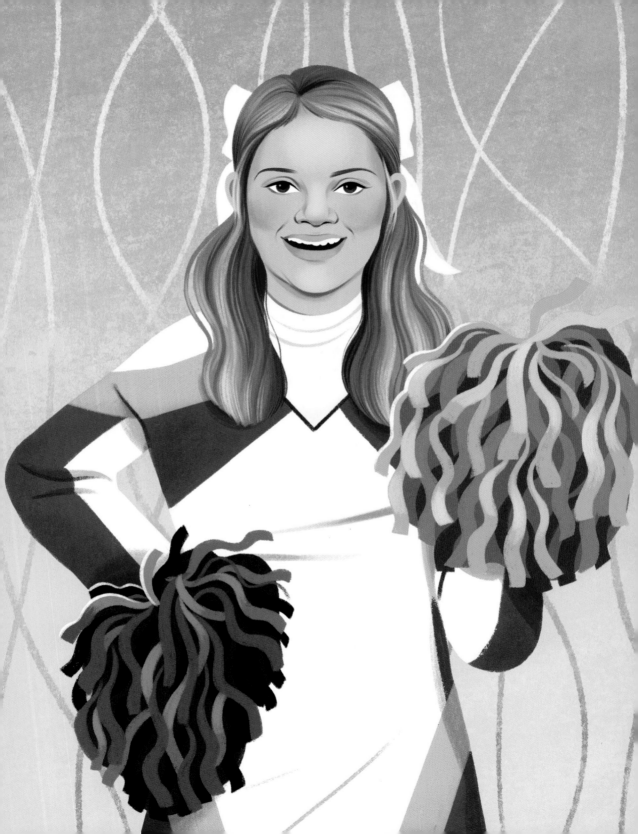

ANNCATHERINE (AC) HEIGL: THE CHEERLEADER

Home Country: The United States • Born in 1998

AnnCatherine Heigl stands at the top of a pyramid of cheerleaders in her green, yellow, and white jersey and short pleated skirt. A big white bow holds back her shoulder-length red hair. As the marching band plays and fans cheer in the stands, she shakes her gold pom-poms above her head and sings her university's fight song:

"Hail to George Mason! Don your Green and Gold!

We're going to sing for George Mason, patriots brave and bold!

We're going to cheer for George Mason, proud for the world to see!

We'll prove our honor and might, and we'll FIGHT! FIGHT! FIGHT!

As we march onward to victory!"

George Mason University's AnnCatherine, who goes by AC, became the first person with Down syndrome to ever cheer on an NCAA Division I team. This is a huge accomplishment, considering university cheerleading is a demanding sport, requiring participants to learn intricate physical routines and chants. They must maintain a high level of energy throughout crowded, noisy athletic events, and always with a smile. This isn't easy, but AC puts her whole heart into cheerleading.

AC grew up in Zionsville, Indiana, with a brother and two sisters. She had several oral surgeries as a child and had to eat only soft foods for a long time. She felt sad that she couldn't eat what her friends at school ate, but she didn't let the disappointment stop her from having fun. AC played competitive tennis with her older sister, Lillie, and then with her younger sister, Mari. She also liked to hang out with her older brother, Tim, and play with their cats and dogs.

While at Zionsville Community High School, AC was a varsity cheerleader and a junior varsity tennis player, and she had numerous friends who loved her sense of humor and bubbly personality. During her freshman and sophomore years, AC's classmates nominated

19

her for homecoming princess. AC loved her French and Spanish clubs and singing in the school choir. She volunteered as a teaching assistant and attended summer camp.

But high school wasn't all fun and games. AC got into occasional arguments with her siblings. She and Lillie shared a bedroom, and when they argued, she'd dump her older sister's belongings from their shared bedroom into the hallway. "I like things to be neat and clean," she explained.

While still in high school, AC watched with envy as Tim and Lillie headed off to college. By her sophomore year, she was asking about her own college visits, eager to attend a university herself. And then the pandemic hit. Like so many other students, AC went to school online. She also did office work at the Chamber of Commerce in Zionsville.

There are very few universities with programs tailored to people with intellectual and developmental disabilities like Down syndrome. So AC applied to George Mason University's elite four-year LIFE program for people with intellectual and developmental disabilities. George Mason University sent AC a letter of acceptance, and she was thrilled. She didn't even mind that she'd be attending college ten hours from her hometown.

AC's family helped her decorate her new dorm room with a pink bedspread, a pillow that read "Sisters Make the Best Friends," and a poster that declared "Life Is Better While Laughing." She tried out for the cheerleading team and won a spot solely based on her talent, dedication, and determination to excel. On the cheerleading team, AC became a flyer, held up in the air by her teammates as she chanted George Mason's fight song. She attended 5:30 a.m. practices and learned all the cheers and dance routines. Her teammates became her close friends, helping her with her makeup and going over cheers with her before big games.

Sadly, AC suffered intense disappointment when she applied to the university's sorority houses. Both her mother and her older sister belonged to sororities, and AC was eager to experience the same sense of belonging and community with a group of sorority sisters. But all eight houses turned her down—a decision Lillie believes was motivated by AC's intellectual and developmental disability.

Still, AC developed self-confidence along with big dreams during her four years at university. Part of her college experience gave her the opportunity to intern on Capitol Hill, helping members of Congress with various administrative tasks.

Postgraduation, AC knew she wanted to stay in the Washington, DC, area for a couple of reasons: Lillie had moved to the area, and AC had become part of a Best Buddies Living program, which allowed her to share an apartment with a former roommate from George Mason. In their apartment, AC enjoys cooking and is particularly skilled at making egg casserole and toast. She also loves crab cakes, mashed potatoes, and Baskin-Robbins daiquiri ice and chocolate ice cream.

With help from Best Buddies, AC found a job at a law firm in DC. She takes public transportation to work, where she handles invoices and emails, prepares documents for mailing, and provides support on various projects. "I have an office job," she says. "I care about being on time, and I care about the people around me."

When she can, AC likes to go out and about. She works out, takes long walks, and hangs out with friends, Lillie, and her future brother-in-law. She loves Taylor Swift, country music, and Christian rock. Preferring happy movies to scary ones, among her favorite films are Disney animated movies, and she has a special fondness for Elsa and her ice powers.

In the future, AC would like to be a cheer coach for kids. In the meantime, she has joined one of her former professors from George Mason as a member of Cheer DC, which is an inclusive organization for any adult who wants to be a cheerleader. "You have to make sure to be on time and show up at practices and all the games," she says. She tells those people hopeful of becoming a flyer on their cheer team, "Don't be scared. But don't fall off."

These words are a motto for the way AC lives her life, with courage and intelligence.

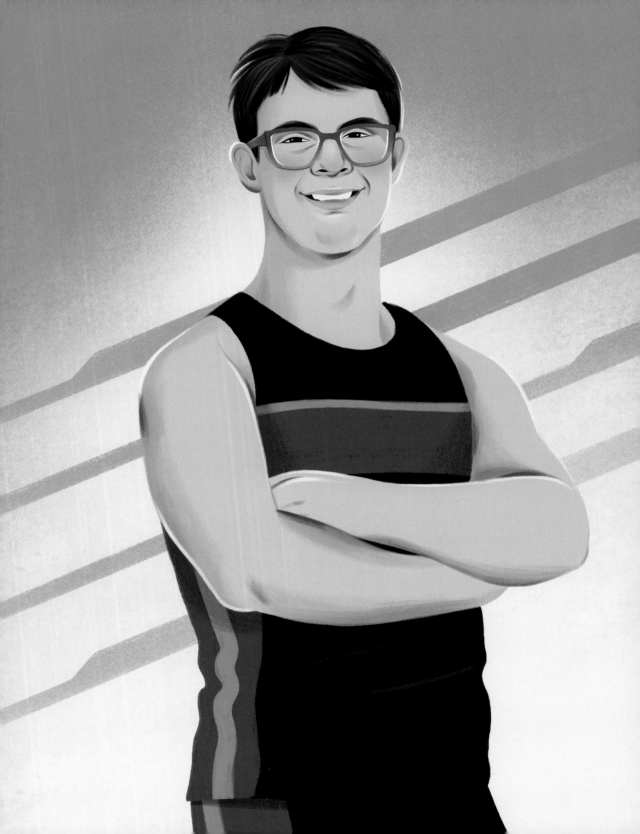

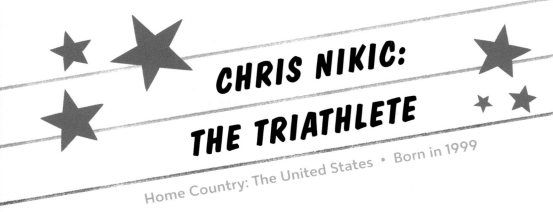

CHRIS NIKIC: THE TRIATHLETE

Home Country: The United States • Born in 1999

During his first Ironman triathlon, Chris Nikic accidentally stepped on a nest of red ants, and they stung him dozens of times. He also swallowed ocean water during the swimming portion of the race and fell off his bike, sustaining an injury so bad that blood ran down his knee. He almost quit during the final leg of the race: a 26.2-mile (marathon-length) run. But his father was right there to help him. "What's going to win, Chris?" his dad asked him. "Your pain or your dreams?"

Chris kept running. And sixteen hours and forty-six minutes after he'd started, he became the first person with Down syndrome to complete an Ironman triathlon.

As a baby, Chris seemed like an unlikely endurance athlete. He had surgery to repair two holes in his heart at five months old. Like many other babies with Down syndrome, he also had small ear canals, which resulted in multiple infections and poor balance. In a photo of Chris at three years old, he's standing up in a walker and grinning at the camera. He didn't learn to walk on his own until he was four years old.

Growing up in Florida, Chris went to seven different elementary schools. He recalls one student calling him *stupid* and *ugly*. He felt isolated and excluded. For a while, his mother homeschooled him. Finally, his parents found a small private school willing to include him. He began to thrive.

At this school, Chris met a best friend, Sam. Together, they played basketball and went to the movies. Chris began to swim, run, and play golf, and when he was sixteen, his parents taught him how to ride a bike. In his first athletic competition, Chris came in last, but he was proud of his medal and well on his way to becoming a triathlete...until he developed problems with his ears.

Suddenly, Chris was homebound with pain and balance issues because of his ears. He had to have multiple surgeries where doctors rebuilt his ear canals. The experience left him weak and unable to swim, even once across a pool. He gained weight. He didn't feel healthy. But Chris was determined to get better. He and his parents found three guides, Carlos, Dan, and Jennifer, who agreed to help Chris train for an Ironman triathlon. Ironman triathalons are races that occur all over the world; participating athletes run 26.2 miles, bike 112 miles, and swim 2.4 miles!

To be a serious competitor, Chris increased his diet to carbs, fruit, vegetables, legumes, lean protein, and lots and lots of water. He became especially fond of Chipotle burrito bowls "with extra beans, extra rice, and extra guacamole," he says.

Chris trained primarily with his dad, but on weekends, he had the support of his three guides from three to five hours daily. Most weekends, he went for hundred-mile bike rides, eighteen-mile runs, and three-mile swims. It was a grueling training schedule, but Chris's dad encouraged him all along the way. He told him to just get one percent better every day.

Chris took that idea to heart. Each day, he did one more lap on his run, in the pool, and on his bike. He did one more squat, one more sit-up, and one more pull-up in the gym. Slowly, he got into shape, and eleven months after he started training, Chris completed the Ironman triathlon in Florida in November 2020. After the event, Chris took a shower, ate a big meal from Waffle House, and had a big party that night with the other athletes. And then suddenly, he became a media star. Reporters from newspapers, magazines, radio, TV, and podcasts wanted to talk with him about his success.

Chris explained that he never saw anyone who looked like him as he was training and completing the Ironman. He wanted to change that. He began a career as an international public speaker, saying people with intellectual and developmental disabilities belong in mainstream competitive sports. He and his father also launched the Runner 321 campaign, which asks race organizers to make a space for people with intellectual and developmental disabilities in every 5K, 10K, half marathon, and marathon run. Chris and his dad also wrote a book together titled *1% Better: Reaching My Full Potential and How You Can Too* and turned it into an illustrated children's book.

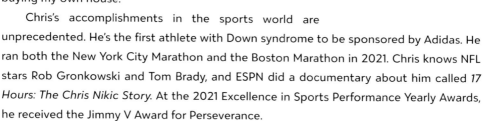

Every day, Chris consults a giant whiteboard in his bedroom. He calls it his Dream Board. He has one big box for his dreams, which inspires him to work hard, and another one labeled "Milestones," where he checks off the races he's completed. On the rest of the board, he writes down his activities for the day—everything from swimming to basketball, from Chipotle lunch to stretching exercises—so that he stays limber for his sports. "I write down my workouts," he says. "And dreams like buying my own house."

Chris's accomplishments in the sports world are unprecedented. He's the first athlete with Down syndrome to be sponsored by Adidas. He ran both the New York City Marathon and the Boston Marathon in 2021. Chris knows NFL stars Rob Gronkowski and Tom Brady, and ESPN did a documentary about him called *17 Hours: The Chris Nikic Story*. At the 2021 Excellence in Sports Performance Yearly Awards, he received the Jimmy V Award for Perseverance.

On his twenty-third birthday in 2022, Chris completed an Ironman in Kona, Hawaii, and in 2023, Chris finished all six World Marathon Majors in New York, Boston, Chicago, Berlin, London, and Tokyo. Marathon Majors take place on famous city streets all over the world, and runners who complete all six earn a coveted Abbott Six Star medal, which Chris now has.

In 2023, the Orlando Magic—Chris's favorite NBA team since he was a child—signed him as a free agent. He received a blue jersey with his name and the number 1 written on the back. The squad welcomed him as an official member.

Chris was particularly excited to play basketball with his favorite Orlando Magic player, power forward Paolo Banchero. In the team's YouTube video documenting Chris's first day with them, an interviewer asks Chris if he has any advice for viewers. Still wearing his official jersey, he looks into the camera and says, "I just want to let them know that each and every person should never give up on a dream."

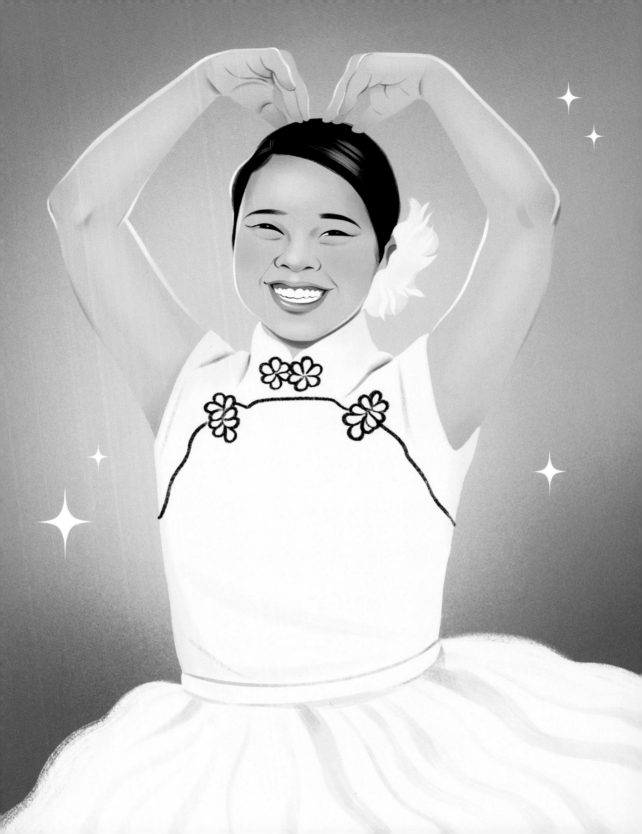

CHRISTINE LAU: THE BALLET DANCER

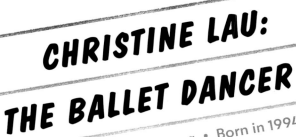

Home Country: Hong Kong • Born in 1994

On an outdoor stage in Hong Kong, surrounded by tall buildings and spectators holding up smartphones, six ballet dancers in white shirts and black tights and skirts move gracefully across the stage, evoking a flock of birds. Suddenly, a young man approaches them with a net in one hand. And then Christine Lau appears center stage wearing a white tutu and black tights, with her long black hair pulled up in a white bow. She begins to dance. Her hands and arms evoke the graceful movements of Odette, the white swan she's portraying in a piece from the classical ballet *Swan Lake*.

Suddenly, Tchaikovsky's serene music morphs into raucous electrical guitars. Christine rips off her tutu, flings it into the audience, and performs a series of leaps and cartwheels. She concludes in a pas de deux that's part dance, part fight scene, with the young man portraying Prince Siegfried and his net. Onlookers stand mesmerized by the grace and power of her performance. At the end of the piece, the other dancers surround Christine, and in a final burst of trumpets, the prince carries her offstage on one shoulder. She waves as people in the audience applaud and cheer.

Christine is a known professional dancer in Hong Kong now, but her path to the spotlight was sometimes rocky. As a child with Down syndrome, it took her four years to learn how to talk. She studied for years with speech and physical therapists to improve her speech and movement. Her parents also enrolled her in ballet classes when she was four, hoping the training would help her build muscle tone and strength. Christine fell in love with ballet's beautiful music and dance moves. She made friends, and ultimately, she found her life's purpose.

Christine has spent her whole life studying ballet, jazz, modern dance, and traditional Chinese dance, which is sometimes performed with a fan or parasol. At first, Christine found ballet difficult. She had to practice every single movement over and over to understand it, and she often fell and ended up bleeding. But she persisted because she wanted to become a professional dancer.

Over the years, Christine recorded each instructor's dance moves and pictured them in her mind, breaking them down into small steps until she could execute each move perfectly. With professional dancers as her teachers, she studied for the Royal Academy of Dance Grade 8 Ballet Examinations. To pass, she had to demonstrate superb posture, body control, and the ability to project emotion through her facial expressions and movements to engage the audience with her performance.

The dancing wasn't the problem. It was the fact that she had to change shoes halfway through the test that proved to be the issue. Like many young dancers, Christine had difficulty tying the ribbons on her ballet shoes tightly enough to stay on her feet. But with hours of practice, she finally mastered the technique and passed her examination.

Christine is part of the Arts with the Disabled Association in Hong Kong, a nonprofit organization that offers opportunities for people with disabilities to excel in the arts and advocate for inclusion through their creative passions. She performs regularly at festivals and competes in dance as well. Christine has a goal of becoming a choreographer.

A nature lover, she's concerned about climate change. Once, she choreographed a dance showing how important it is to protect the environment, scattering plastic bags across the stage and dancing through them to show how plastic is harming the earth.

In 2014, Christine represented Hong Kong in the Pyeongchang Special Music and Art Festival in Korea. In 2015, the Australian Teachers of Dancing certified that Christine had successfully passed the standard required by the Gold Medal Jazz Moves examination. She then traveled to Bordeaux, France, in 2016 to perform in the Ninth International Abilympics. And in 2019, she became the first person with a disability to receive the distinguished award CCDC Dance Laureate from the City Contemporary Dance Hong Kong. The award goes to people who've made powerful contributions to contemporary dance in the region.

Today, Christine works as a teaching assistant for dance groups at the Hong Kong Down Syndrome Association, and she's a jazz dance assistant at the school she attended as a child. Her accomplishments are significant because in Hong Kong, very few dancers with Down syndrome find work as professional performers and educators. More typically, they work as office assistants or janitors. In 2023, *Tatler Asia*, a luxury lifestyle magazine, featured Christine on its magazine cover and profiled her as a role model among the approximately three thousand people with Down syndrome in Hong Kong.

When she isn't dancing or teaching, Christine likes to spend time with her mother and father and go hiking. "In Hong Kong, we have a lot of beautiful mountains," she says. Her father often bakes homemade bread for her, which she has with her power breakfast of eggs and a glass of milk to keep up her strength for dancing. She loves listening to music too, especially beautiful classical pieces.

In the future, Christine wants to keep dancing and teaching so she can share her knowledge with others. "Through teaching, I build up my confidence as a dancer, and I enjoy seeing students engaging passionately with the dancing," she says. Some of her students are people with intellectual and developmental disabilities. "It can be challenging to help them control their emotions and to make sure they're listening to my instructions," she says, "but I love teaching. I want to try my best to make a contribution to the community, and I'll help others to make a contribution to the community as well," she explains.

Christine likes to remind people that everyone has different abilities and different kinds of strength. "We have to enjoy our life," she says, "and engage in the world with passion."

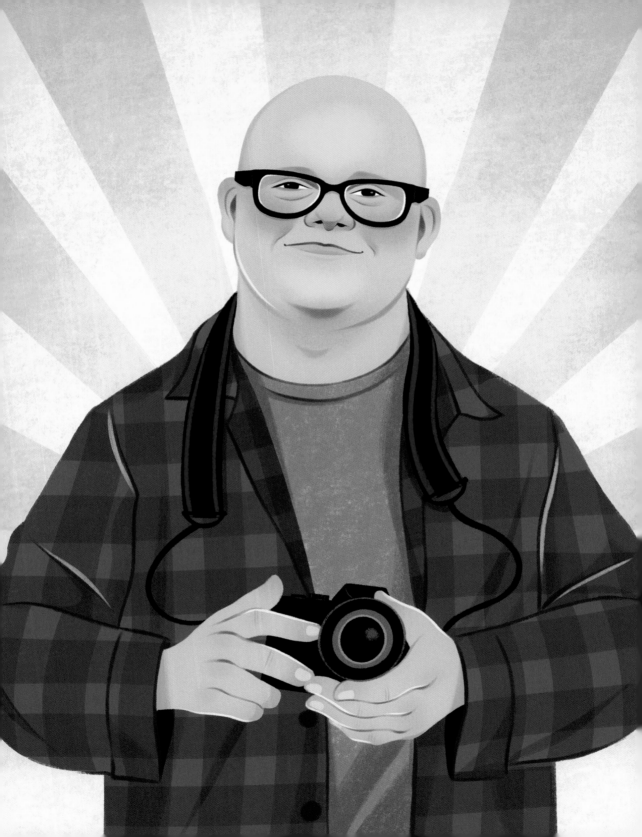

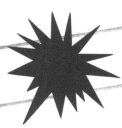

GEOFFREY MIKOL: THE PHOTOGRAPHER

Home Country: The United States • Born in 1994

Geoffrey Mikol discovered his life's work one day in high school when his teacher, Mr. Seymour, asked students to take photographs and bring them to class. Mr. Seymour saw Geoffrey's images and told his mother her son's way of capturing light in his photos was "extraordinary." One of Geoffrey's earliest photographs, titled "First Light," shows early morning sunlight streaming through trees in a field full of flowers. It's a magical image.

"Photography is awesome and cool," Geoffrey says before adding that he particularly likes to capture spooky images, as in his photograph titled "Vanishing Tracks." It shows a railroad track disappearing into trees, surrounded by eerie fog.

Because of Geoffrey's clear passion for photography, his mother bought him a Nikon camera while he was still in high school, and he began walking the streets of Washington, DC, searching for subjects to photograph. Mr. Seymour mentored Geoffrey during all four years of high school, teaching him about light, focus, and how to develop prints in a darkroom.

Geoffrey's high school attracted students from all over the world because there were all kinds of government officials from different countries who lived near Washington, DC. As part of this diverse community in high school, Geoffrey felt valued and respected. He played basketball with Special Olympics and acted in community theater. "I loved to play villains," he says and flexes his impressive biceps.

Geoffrey also got involved with his high school's Best Buddies program, and he made a lot of friends. On the last day of his senior year, his teachers threw him a party, and students from all four grades attended. His classroom got so crowded that the teachers had to move the party outside! Geoffrey ended up standing on the table to give a goodbye speech, surrounded by hundreds of his friends.

Geoffrey thrived in college as well, especially in his job in the mail room and his

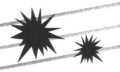

cooking classes, where he learned to make homemade pasta sauce, hash browns, eggs, and his specialty, shepherd's pie. But his passion continued to be landscape photography. Geoffrey took pictures of trees, rocks, old barns, waterfalls, and flowers, appreciating the play of light and shadows on objects on rural roads and in state and national parks.

After college, Geoffrey began exhibiting his work in juried art shows in the Chicago area, where he won several awards for his photography. His work was well received. So in January 2016, Geoffrey, his dad, and his stepmom moved to Galena, Illinois, to open his gallery, called River Bend. His mom followed shortly after. Geoffrey became very popular, and his business grew so much that the gallery was moved to a larger location on Main Street.

Galena is a tourist town about three hours west of Chicago that gets about 1.5 million visitors a year from all over the U.S. and the world. Geoffrey applied for and was named an "Illinois Maker" by the State of Illinois Tourism Board in 2019. Geoffrey's business was also awarded Business of the Year in 2019 by the Galena Chamber of Commerce. Geoffrey has had multiple articles written about him, he has been a guest speaker at events, and NBC News interviewed him about his gallery and art. His photographs were also exhibited at the fiftieth anniversary of the World Special Olympics.

Geoffrey is always looking for things to photograph, even when in a car with his dad or mom. If he sees something, he tells them to "stop, this is it!" so he can get out and take a photo. One of those photos became "Quiet Swing," which shows a bench swing overlooking a peaceful river. Another is "Dark Rocks," a configuration of boulders in water that creates a heart-shaped pool.

Geoffrey is always thinking about new ways to display his photographs. One winter, he looked up from the dinner table. "I have an idea," he told his family. "Snow globes! Who doesn't like a snow globe?" Besides framed photographs, Geoffrey's photos are displayed in multiple mediums including metal, reclaimed barnwood, and items like coasters, note cards, and puzzles. All his items are for sale both online and in his gallery, and they are produced in the family's studio.

At the gallery, Geoffrey likes to talk with visitors about his work and helps to box up purchases and prepare new items for sale. The gallery can get crowded, and customers want to ask Geoffrey questions and pose with him for selfies. Sometimes it can be overwhelming. But he loves meeting people, especially fellow sports fans of his two favorite teams: the Chicago Cubs and the Chicago Bears.

In his free time, Geoffrey walks around Galena taking photographs. He and his family also travel in search of new landscapes. In Colorado, he shot "One Buck," a photo of an elk looking straight into the camera. He also caught a close-up shot of a monarch butterfly on a flower, leaning close in and staying perfectly still even though honeybees swarmed around him. "That was scary," he admits. "When I was younger, a wasp flew in my ear."

These days, Geoffrey listens to Blake Shelton, Luke Bryan, and Maroon 5. He watches *The Voice*, scary movies, and the Cubs and Bears. He also developed a love of dogs and country music. "I'm a country boy," he says. He loves getting together with his friends to hang out and talk or play games such as trivia. He also likes to spend time with his parents and his dog, Tiger.

In the future, Geoffrey would like to teach music to preschool students. He's thrilled to be an uncle to his stepbrother's little girl. He'd also like to travel to the Grand Canyon and the Badlands to study the landscapes and take new photographs.

His words for those who might be curious about people with Down syndrome? "We are awesome and cool."

His suggestions for those who might want to get started in photography? "Just go out and walk and take pictures of what you see. Practice as much as you can."

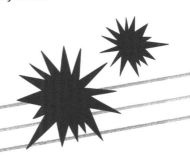

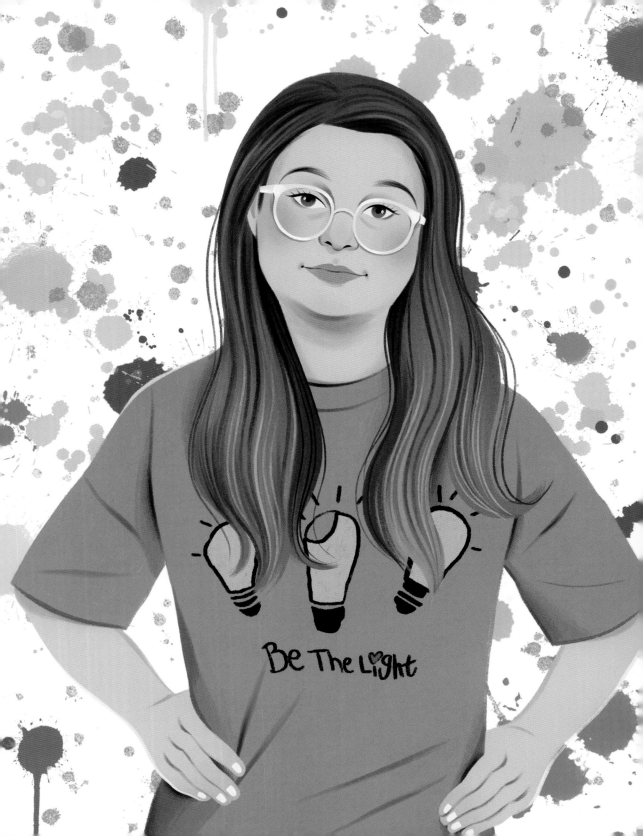

GRACE KEY: THE ARTIST

Home Country: The United States • Born in 1998

Grace Key loves to have what she calls "Chit Chats" on Instagram and TikTok. During one midsummer chat, she sat in the passenger seat of her mother's car with her long brown hair in a ponytail and a blue tank top decorated with an image of the earth surrounded by hearts. When her mother asked her to offer her 334K followers one piece of advice to be happy in life, Grace looked into the camera and said, "Come and party with me!" And then she burst out laughing.

Grace lives in Calhoun, Georgia. She is the founder of Candidly Kind, a T-shirt and apparel company she started with her mother on World Down Syndrome Day in 2018 to showcase her witty catchphrases and colorful works of art. She grew up painting, drawing, and writing creatively to express her emotions. She's naturally upbeat and prefers to call her genetic condition "Up Syndrome." However, as she points out in a Facebook post, "People with Down Syndrome are not always happy. I'm usually happy, but I do get mad and sad."

For example, she felt both angry and sad as an honorary high school cheerleader when her coach wouldn't let her on the field with the rest of her squad during the football game. Grace could only cheer from the other side of a fence, separated from the other cheerleaders. She wasn't allowed to ride the bus to away games either. Her sister wrote about these incidents on Facebook. People in their small town became so outraged that they circulated a petition to allow Grace to cheer with her squad. They collected five thousand signatures, and the school district apologized to Grace.

The next year, however, both the coach and most of the other cheerleaders began to bully her. So Grace quit the squad and focused on art, including T-shirt designs, in her last year of high school instead. Her art teacher helped her with her first T-shirt design: three bright yellow light bulbs to illustrate her advice to "be the light." Her family helped her to print up a few hundred shirts and launch Candidly Kind using the internet and social media. She sold almost half the shirts she had printed during her first week of business.

Now Grace offers dozens of designs on hoodies, tote bags, onesies, stickers, and, of course, T-shirts. During the pandemic, she created face masks with her designs and donated one hundred percent of the sales to a hospital in Atlanta. One woman who worked there was so captivated by Grace's designs that she purchased seventy-five masks.

Grace paints her designs at a table surrounded by her whimsical artwork. She's got brushes in every shape and size and boxes full of colorful paints. When she's not painting for her business, she creates labels and cleverly packages her T-shirts and hats, including a handwritten thank-you note to every customer. Sometimes she stays up most of the night writing them.

Grace ships her products to every U.S. state and to twenty-two countries. Her local boutique carries her T-shirts as well, each one with her handmade label that reads "Look what I made! T-shirts designed by Grace Key, Candidly Kind," and includes a line drawing of her. She's donated a percentage of every sale—totaling thousands of dollars—to her favorite charities, including Ruby's Rainbow, which gives scholarships to adults with Down syndrome to help them attend college.

Grace also has a passion for makeup. She loves watching makeup tutorials and began creating videos of her own on social media, showing how she applies makeup. Staff at the cosmetics company Urban Decay saw her posts and hired her to do digital content creation for the brand. In one Instagram video, Grace demonstrates how to apply blush and highlighter from the company; in another, she shows viewers how to use a bright blue eyeliner pencil. "I create the campaigns, and my mom does all the editing," she explains. The lifestyle box brand FabFitFun has featured Grace in a TV commercial and in their online advertising.

Grace has taken classes in advocacy training so that she can articulate her needs and the needs of her peers with Down syndrome. In a speech to the Down Syndrome Association of Atlanta, she pointed out that she and others deserve to work for competitive wages. She explained that people with Down syndrome are dependable and they work hard.

Grace has also given keynotes at the annual Dear Mom, Conference, which brings together mothers who have children with Down syndrome at a one-day event where they meet one another and learn from guest speakers. Grace likes to open her keynote presentations with these words: "Hey, party people! I own a business!"

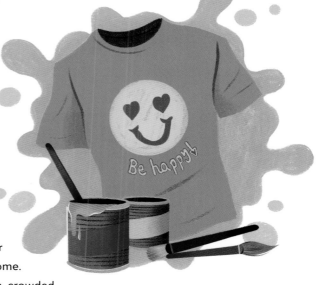

In 2022, she appeared on *Fox and Friends* with Hawaiian shirt designer Nate Simon, who also has Down syndrome. They stood with reporters at a table in crowded Fox Square on Sixth Avenue in New York City and spoke about their products. Grace displayed her framed artwork as well as many of her T-shirt designs, including one of her favorites: dark blue printed with the words "Hey Party People!" When asked about the message she wanted to spread by starting Candidly Kind, she told the reporter, "I want to spread awareness, kindness, and love and shine a light."

The best part of her job is "making people smile," Grace says. The most difficult part is getting to the post office each day before it closes to mail out her orders to customers. Fortunately, she's got friends at the post office who help her out if she's a bit late. In 2023, Gigi's Playhouse Atlanta gave Candidly Kind the SKate Award, recognizing Grace's service to humanity through her artwork and her advocacy.

In her free time, Grace loves to hang out with her family and friends and her big brown boxer, Ellie Mae. Grace watches college football on TV and roots for the Clemson Tigers from South Carolina. She enjoys hamburgers from Freddy's Frozen Custard and Steakburgers, so much so that she designed a shirt with an illustration of a burger, fries, and ketchup above the words "Eat more burgers." She adores dressing up and dancing... often to Bruno Mars. You'll always find Grace in the middle of the party!

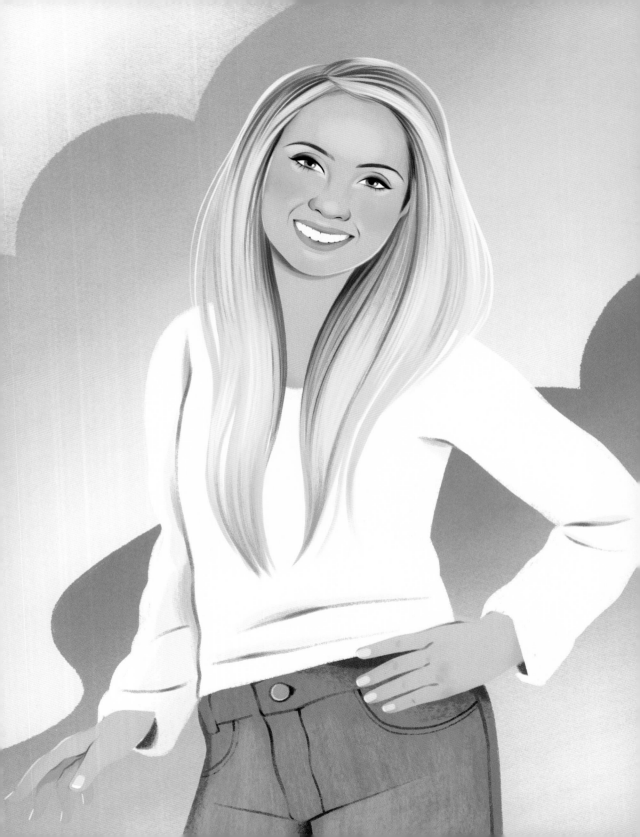

GRACE STROBEL: THE JOY CREATOR

Home Country: The United States • Born in 1996

Grace Strobel remembers her first job in the lunchroom at the school she'd once attended in St. Louis, Missouri. She was just twenty years old. She loved helping kids and feeling a sense of belonging. One day, a group of kids asked for help opening their fruit cups and milk cartons. Grace struggled with the task. Then she looked up and realized they were making fun of her. Devastated, she ran to the kitchen and burst into tears.

She felt scared and alone, the victim of hatred. She went home and told her mother what had happened. Grace cried on her bed for four days, feeling worthless and lonely. Her mother realized the kids were reacting out of fear; perhaps they had never seen someone with Down syndrome before. "What do you want to do about this?" her mother asked her.

This was not the first time Grace had to navigate challenges. When she was born, doctors told her parents that she'd never be able to read or tie her shoes and that there was no shame in putting her in an institution. Her parents were outraged. They brought their little girl home and learned how to help her strengthen her body. Grace was homeschooled until she was eight years old. After she entered public school, she did extra academic assignments at home because teachers would give her coloring sheets instead of giving her the same work they gave her classmates.

When Grace was in middle school, she and her mother went to a presentation by Karen Gaffney (see page 62), a professional speaker and the first swimmer with Down syndrome to complete a relay swim across the English Channel. Grace was impressed with Karen's accomplishments and left feeling inspired and motivated. When Grace graduated from high school, she found a job in the elementary school she'd attended.

But after the bullying incident in the lunchroom, Grace decided to create a presentation called "The Grace Effect" and take it around to schools with the help of her mother. They hoped to change people's perceptions of those with disabilities, inform them of

Grace's particular challenges, and teach the importance of showing kindness and respect to all kinds of people.

First, Grace set to work researching Down syndrome. After two months of daily research, she learned a lot, including that people with her genetic condition often have low muscle tone and need to work harder to accomplish tasks that require both fine and gross motor skills. She and her mother came up with role-playing activities to demonstrate the various challenges people with Down syndrome deal with daily:

To show how low muscle tone impedes the body's ability to move quickly, Grace asks kids to sit in a beanbag chair wearing a heavy backpack and then try to stand up.

To show how tasks requiring fine motor skills can be difficult, she asks kids to put on mittens and then attempt to button their coats.

To demonstrate the low vision of some people with Down syndrome, she asks them to look through unfocused binoculars.

To demonstrate how balance can be a struggle, she has kids walk on BOSU balls.

Finally, she tells kids that making fun of someone lasts a few seconds...but the pain this causes can last a lifetime. "It hurts me to see someone not included," she says. "No matter who you are, we all want to be valued and respected and to feel good about ourselves."

Grace has given her presentation to thousands of students in and around St. Louis. Each time she speaks, kids crowd around her for hugs and high fives. They send her thank-you letters and tell her that she's taught them so much. She's a role model and an inspiration to teachers as well. "Down syndrome is not a bad or scary thing," she says. "I am very typical—it just takes me longer to do things. I have a great life with career, friends, and family."

Grace loved her work as a presenter, but she wanted more. During her research into people with Down syndrome, she saw a photo of supermodel Madeline Stuart, who has the genetic condition too. Grace asked her parents if she might become a model, so they hired a professional photographer and posted Grace's photos on Facebook. The photos went viral, and suddenly, she found herself with a modeling career.

As a model, Grace has walked the New York Fashion Week runway for Tommy Hilfiger Adaptive, and she's partnered with skincare line Obagi and the clothing brand Alivia. She's a rep for Rihanna's line of skincare products called Fenty Beauty, and she even posed with Rihanna for a picture at a Hollywood party. Modeling makes Grace feel good about herself and helps other people with disabilities to believe in themselves and their dreams.

As a public personality, Grace uses her Instagram and TikTok accounts to lift up people with disabilities. In one of her posts, she highlights many of those represented in this book. "We are pretty cool people to hang out with," she says. "Why not try it yourself!"

In her free time, Grace runs three miles a day and works out at the gym. She participates in 5K races with her mother and competes on her Special Olympics track and field team. She loves to dance and listen to music; one of her favorite singers is Bruno Mars. She also hangs out with her friends, cooks, and watches movies. She loves the *Harry Potter* films and especially Hermione Granger because she's so smart.

Grace looks forward to many more years of modeling and public speaking. She's eager to break down barriers for people and inspire them to achieve their goals while practicing kindness.

"Believe in yourself. You can make a difference in the world. Speak up when you see something wrong. Never give up. Sometimes our biggest sorrows become our greatest achievements."

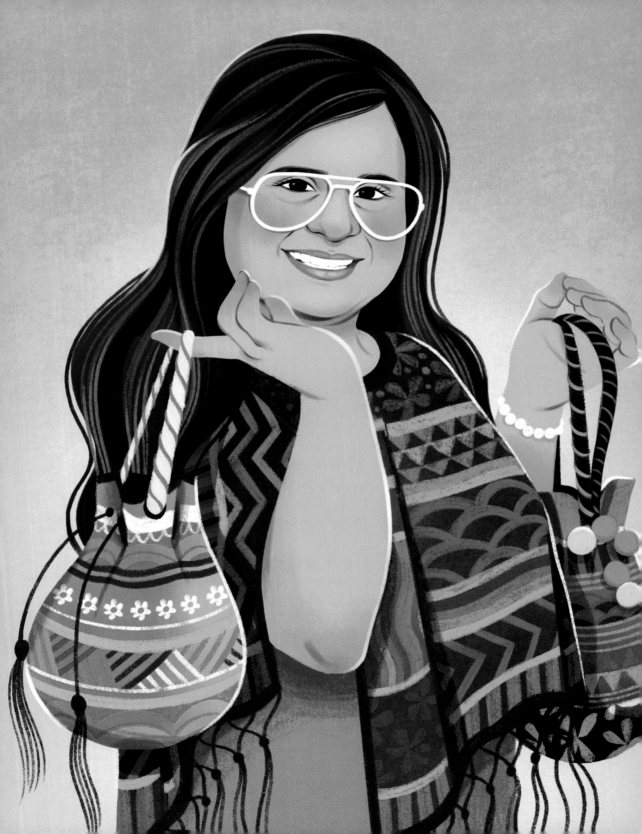

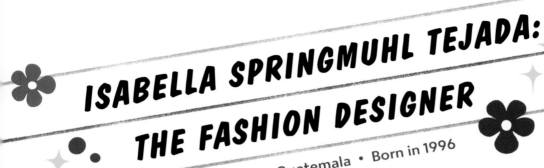

ISABELLA SPRINGMUHL TEJADA: THE FASHION DESIGNER

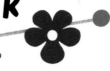

Home Country: Guatemala • Born in 1996

Isabella Springmuhl Tejada grew up the youngest of four children in a sewing studio in Guatemala City. Her grandmother designed clothes using traditional Guatemalan textiles and sold them in a boutique called Xjabelle. As a child, Isabella read fashion magazines and sketched outfits for her dolls on paper. Then she began sewing clothes from scraps of her grandmother's fabric. Little did anyone know that soon, she'd have a boutique of her own!

Isabella's mother nicknamed her Belita, which means "little beauty." Isabella had long brown hair, brown eyes, and a sweet smile. Still, she struggled to make friends in school. The other kids thought Down syndrome was a type of disease, and they wouldn't hang out with her. Finally, she and her mother created a book to explain Down syndrome. It worked, and in high school, Isabella's friends chose her to give their graduation farewell speech.

Isabella loved clothes, but growing up, she couldn't find any that fit her body type. People with Down syndrome often have shorter-than-average torsos, necks, arms, and legs. Pants, shirts, skirts, and dresses were either too long or too short on Isabella. Her mother constantly had to alter her clothing.

Isabella had a dream of making clothes that actually fit people with Down syndrome, so when she graduated from college, she decided to become a fashion designer. She applied to fashion schools in Guatemala, but the teachers worried that she wouldn't be able to handle the demanding curriculum because she had Down syndrome. They told her no.

"I felt devastated," Isabella says. "My whole life, my family, friends, and teachers had told me I could do anything I wanted. I felt like my dreams had crumbled."

But Isabella did not give up. Her mother enrolled her in a dressmaking academy where she learned to embroider, create paper patterns, and use a sewing machine. She found a way to turn a *no* into a *yes.*

In the dressmaking academy, Isabella designed a handbag inspired by the woven textile *tzutes* that indigenous Mayan women fold around their fruits and vegetables at the market and then balance on their heads as they walk back home.

One sewing teacher asked Isabella to design clothing for tiny handmade figures called "worry dolls," which children in Guatemala and Mexico put under their pillows. Instead, Isabella made human-size dolls and outfitted them in multicolored embroidered ponchos and jackets made from brightly woven textiles. These pieces foreshadowed her future success as a clothing designer.

When Isabella's grandmother died, she left behind her clothing design studio. Isabella's family helped her to launch Down to Xjabelle, an inclusive clothing and accessory brand featuring vibrant fabrics and embroidered designs. She's inspired by the patterns, textures, and colors of Guatemala with its rich history of weaving and using textiles as a way of storytelling. She chooses and purchases her textiles from Mayan indigenous women who work in Guatemala's rural regions. The weavers use individual patterns and colors according to their region. A group of people with physical and developmental disabilities makes the beadwork that Isabella incorporates into her designs. She pays everyone fair wages, and she's committed to showcasing the handwork of people from underrepresented communities.

Isabella designs clothes for all body types. In a studio packed with textiles and baskets of colored embroidery thread, Isabella first draws the designs for new clothes and then colors them in. She uses special software to create 3D printouts, then sends the patterns to a workshop where seamstresses and embroiderers create each piece of clothing. Often, Isabella adds beads, tassels, fringes, and pom-poms to her pieces. People from all over the world order her one-of-a-kind clothes through Instagram.

In 2015, Guatemala's Ixchel Museum of Indigenous Textiles and Clothing invited Isabella to showcase her designs, and she sold out her collection. In 2016, Isabella became the first designer with Down syndrome invited to showcase her creations at London Fashion Week—and to huge applause. That year, the BBC included her on its list of one hundred inspirational women of 2016. At first, Isabella was afraid to travel to London; she didn't know how people would treat her as a Guatemalan woman with Down syndrome, but she was thrilled to find that people were kind to her.

In 2019, Isabella displayed one of her clothing collections at All Inclusive Runway in Mexico City, which featured nineteen models, eleven of whom had a disability. One of her models was Paralympic athlete Michel Muñoz Malagón, born without legs, who modeled with a skateboard while wearing a denim jacket that Isabella designed. It was embellished with black fringe, colorfully embroidered stripes and shapes, and sleeve cuffs with traditional textiles.

At the All Inclusive Runway, she met Mexican actor Francisco "Paco" de la Fuente who'd traveled there to meet her. The two fell in love. Now they talk every evening on FaceTime and plan to get married. "I'm going to design my own wedding dress," Isabella says. "I want to look like a Greek goddess."

In 2023, Isabella debuted a line of dresses and saris that incorporated traditional Indian textiles along with Guatemalan fabrics to celebrate the twenty-fifth anniversary of Fundación Margarita Tejada, the school Isabella's family founded for people with Down syndrome. "I love designing beautiful dresses like the ones on Disney princesses," she explains, adding that Elsa and Merida are her favorites.

When she's not designing clothing or speaking internationally, Isabella takes opera singing lessons inspired by her grandfather. She loves the operas *Turandot, La Bohème,* and anything by Puccini. She likes to dance, ride horses, play tennis, and do Zumba, both as a student and as a teacher. She wants to inspire other people with disabilities and teach them how to, as she says, "change a no to a yes."

"People with Down syndrome are able to achieve their dreams, work, and become entrepreneurs," Isabella says. "It's normal to have obstacles, but we can achieve our dreams."

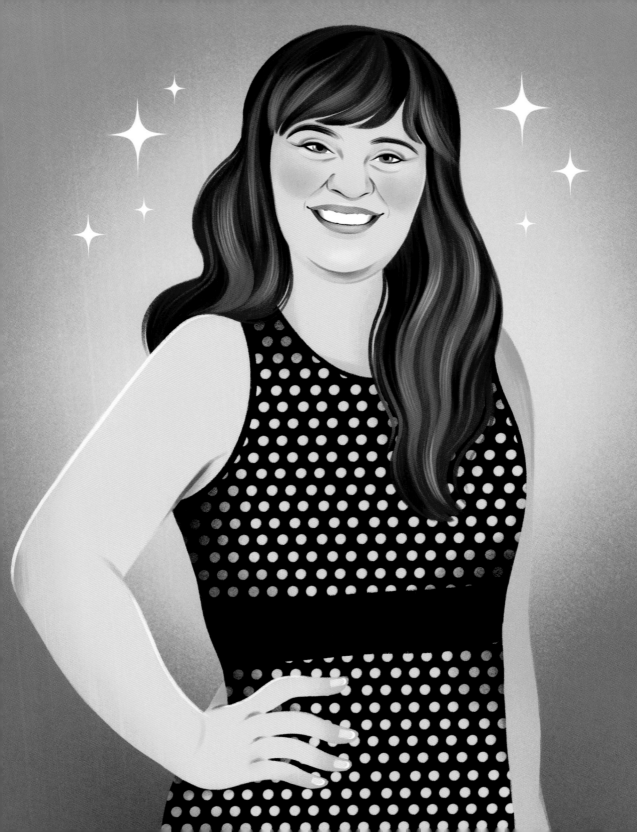

JAMIE BREWER: THE ACTOR

Home Country: The United States • Born in 1985

When Jamie Brewer was growing up in Southern California and Houston, Texas, she loved going to movies and attending live theater performances. When she saw Chris Burke, an actor with Down syndrome, in the TV series *Life Goes On,* she was inspired by him.

Jamie was fully included in all her classrooms from kindergarten through high school, and in eighth grade, she began to take theater classes. As a middle schooler, she was outgoing and energetic. "I was really into schoolwork," she says. Later, she trained in Houston's Dionysus Theater, which includes actors both with and without disabilities, studying drama, comedy, and improvisation. She studied acting and learned about the entertainment industry in college.

Jamie booked the first audition she went on, landing a role as Addie Langdon in the popular TV series *American Horror Story* (TV-MA). Addie is a curious girl who is friends with ghosts. Jamie also played a mind-reading witch in the third season and a ventriloquist's doll who comes to life in the fourth season. Jamie appeared at the Emmy Awards several times, stopping on the red carpet in gorgeous gowns to talk about the importance of inclusion and disability rights.

In 2018, Jamie became the first model with Down syndrome to walk the catwalk in New York Fashion Week for designer Carrie Hammer's show called "Role Models Not Runway Models." Jamie wore a designer belted V-neck dress and bright red lipstick, walking down the runway to the beat of Fifth Harmony's song "Worth It." She radiated confidence as she smiled at the audience, knowing she'd just expanded the way society thinks about beauty.

Jamie has starred in several short films and in a music video. She played a soon-to-be bride who worries about her brother's strange behavior in the comedy *Whitney's Wedding.* She starred in the comedy film *Turnover,* and she appeared with Zack Gottsagen (see page

102) in rock band Delta Spirit's music video "What's Done Is Done." In it, she's a woman in her eighties who falls back in love with her husband after she recalls their first years as a couple.

In her early thirties, Jamie became the first woman with Down syndrome to star in an off-Broadway play. She appeared in *Amy and the Orphans,* the story of three adult siblings who come together to deal with the death of their father. Her character spent most of her life in group homes, and she challenges her older brother and sister to see her as a person rather than a disability. Jamie won the Drama Desk Award for Outstanding Featured Actress in a Play for her work. When people ask her whether she prefers acting onstage or on-screen, she says "Both. I've been a theater girl my whole life, and I love all of it."

Jamie also appeared in the world premiere of the play *Corsicana.* Written by Will Arbery, whose sister has Down syndrome, it's the story of two siblings who've lost their mother and deal with grief while figuring out how to take care of each other. Jamie plays Ginny, the outspoken older sister, and gets to dance and sing onstage. While rehearsing for the role, Jamie would sometimes use sign language as well as speech. The practice helped her to memorize all her lines. She uses a variety of methods to warm up her voice before acting and singing; one of her favorites is to talk in an extremely high-pitched tone. "I'm a natural alto," she says, "but when I talk in a high soprano like Alvin and the Chipmunks, it helps my voice to resonate later when I'm performing."

In 2015, the Global Down Syndrome Foundation awarded Jamie the Quincy Jones Exceptional Advocacy Award for her work as a humanitarian who strives to change the public's perception of people with Down syndrome and to end discrimination and bigotry. In a 2018 video she made for Special Olympics, Jamie says, "Don't let disability hold you back, no matter what. Use your disability to an advantage."

Jamie has been a tireless participant in the Spread the Word to End the Word campaign, which asks communities and schools to publicly pledge their support of people with intellectual and developmental disabilities. As part of the

Governmental Affairs Committee of The Arc of Texas, which serves people with intellectual and developmental disabilities, Jamie helped persuade her Texas state representatives to abolish the word *retard* from government documents and use the term *intellectual or developmental disability* instead. In 2018, she spoke to *The Today Show*, explaining that if she hears someone using the r-word—even if they're just teasing someone—she tells them kindly but firmly that their words are hurtful, and they need to stop.

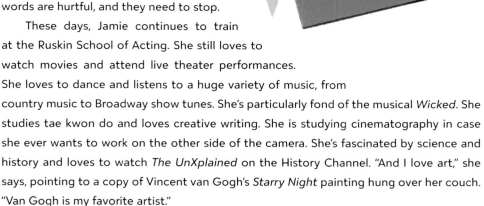

These days, Jamie continues to train at the Ruskin School of Acting. She still loves to watch movies and attend live theater performances. She loves to dance and listens to a huge variety of music, from country music to Broadway show tunes. She's particularly fond of the musical *Wicked*. She studies tae kwon do and loves creative writing. She is studying cinematography in case she ever wants to work on the other side of the camera. She's fascinated by science and history and loves to watch *The UnXplained* on the History Channel. "And I love art," she says, pointing to a copy of Vincent van Gogh's *Starry Night* painting hung over her couch. "Van Gogh is my favorite artist."

Jamie has been an inspirational speaker for numerous international organizations that advocate for the rights of people with Down syndrome and other disabilities. She's on the board of directors for the Down Syndrome Association of Orange County. "We work behind the scenes organizing golf tournaments and other fundraising events," she says. In the video she made for Special Olympics in 2018, Jamie tells people, "Never give up. Don't see yourself with your disability. Don't label yourself, and never, never give up."

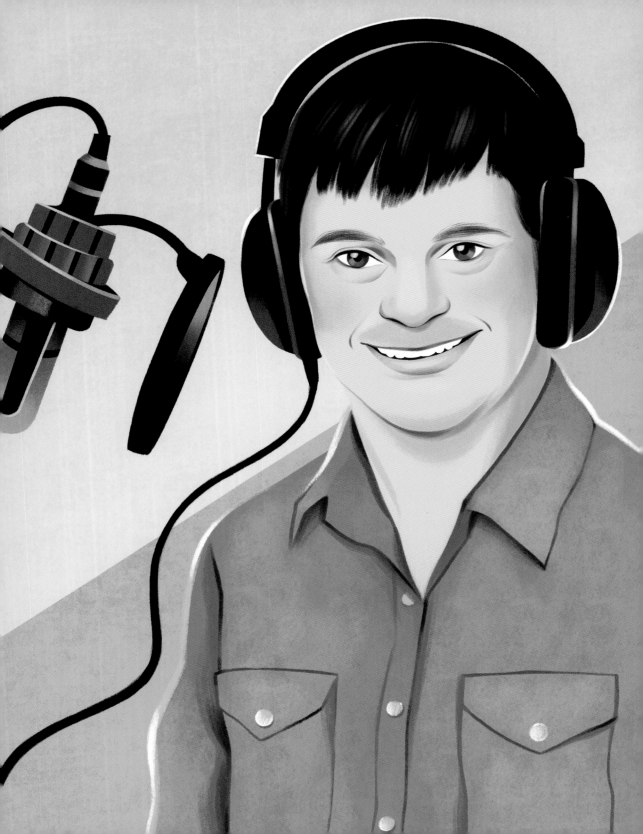

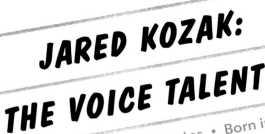

JARED KOZAK: THE VOICE TALENT

Home Country: The United States • Born in 1989

I f you've ever watched Nickelodeon's shows *The Loud House* and *The Casagrandes,* you know the character C.J. He's the second-oldest child in his family, a fun-loving kid, and an expert hairstylist who happens to have Down syndrome. He's voiced by Jared Kozak, Nickelodeon's first-ever voice-over talent with Down syndrome.

Jared grew up in Southern California with his younger brother, Jeremy, and he was fully included in regular classrooms from kindergarten through college. If someone bullied Jared's shy little brother on the playground, Jared would stick up for him, and the bully always apologized.

Jared has an excellent sense of humor; he loves to joke around and says Robin Williams is his favorite actor and comedian of all time. He grew up reading sports-themed books and magazines as well as *Scooby Doo* and *Avengers* comics. His favorite author is football player and writer Tim Tebow, and his favorite movies are the *Harry Potter* films, which he's also listened to as audiobooks. Jared's bedroom walls are decorated with posters for the Las Vegas Raiders, the Los Angeles Rams, and the Washington Capitals.

Jared has competed in Special Olympics since he was eleven, focusing on basketball, bowling, and golf. He's a Special Olympics Global Messenger, responsible for giving presentations to companies and schools all over Los Angeles and Orange County. "I get people to donate money and sign up to volunteer for Special Olympics," he says proudly.

In middle school and high school, Jared worked in the school cafeteria. He also managed the boys' varsity basketball team all four years of high school and had his own column, called "Kozak's Korner," in his school newspaper. The column showcased his interviews with athletes and coaches. "Kids with disabilities should be with regular kids at school and not in a room by themselves," he says.

Jared attended Fullerton College for four years and majored in acting. He learned to slow down his speaking and help with his stutter, at least most of the time. "It's okay to breathe regularly," he says about the process of delivering his lines.

As a college student, Jared did a report on journalist Geraldo Rivera who, in 1972, took a camera crew to Willowbrook State School in Staten Island, New York, and showed the world how children with disabilities were being abused. "A long time ago, they would put kids in this room and discriminate against them," Jared explains. "Geraldo came in and said, 'This is not right. Put them in a regular school.' It opened people's eyes, and they put those kids in a regular school."

Later, Jared became friends with actor Luke Spinelli; they appeared together in *Leader of the Pack*, a 2012 web series about a girl who wants to save the world and falls in love with a boy who has Down syndrome. The role marked Jared's first job as a professional actor. "I love acting," he says, "and I have appeared in many independent films."

Jared has acted in the films *Orson's Last Dance, Y'all-R Family*, and *Goodbye Dessa*. He's also had a recurring role as a hospital volunteer on the soap opera *General Hospital*. But his main job is voicing C.J. for the Nickelodeon shows *The Loud House* and its spin-off, *The Casagrandes,* which aired for three seasons and already won two Emmys. In 2023, a Netflix movie for *The Casagrandes* was in production.

Before COVID-19, Jared went to the studio to record his lines. During and after the pandemic, he recorded in his parents' walk-in closet with the script in front of him while talking with his director on the computer. "The director will tell me how she wants me to say the lines," he says. "Sometimes I have to say the line six or seven times because she wants it right-on perfect."

In 2021, Jared had the chance to design a pair of cleats for Los Angeles Rams player Johnny Hekker. Both men participated in the My Cause My Cleats program, which lets the public know about different philanthropic organizations. Jared came up with a red, gold, and blue design that included the Special Olympics logo and the phrase "Hugs and Smiles" on one cleat and "Brave in the Attempt" on the other. Johnny wore the cleats on the day Jared attended one of his football games.

That same year, Jared was the Celebrity Grand Marshal in Whittier, California's sixty-seventh annual Christmas parade. Sporting a bright red shirt and a Christmas-themed tie, he stood up and waved at crowds of people from a cherry-red antique car.

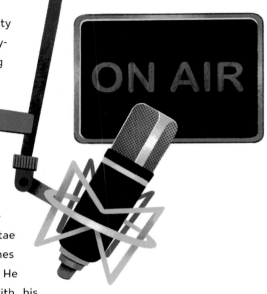

These days, when he's not working as an actor or voice talent, Jared is an usher at the La Mirada Theater in Southern California. He takes classes in acting, hip-hop, and jazz dancing, does yoga and tae kwon do, goes to the movies, and watches sports—especially when USC is playing. He loves attending backyard barbecues with his family and friends, and he enjoys eating Chinese food—particularly honey walnut shrimp—and singing karaoke.

"We are more alike than different," he says of people with Down syndrome, borrowing a line he spoke in *Orson's Last Dance*. "Sometimes it takes us a little more time to learn something," he adds, "but really, we can do almost anything."

In the future, Jared would like to work with a sports team and star in a feature film. He's devoted to continuing to work for inclusion too. "I would like to see everyone be included no matter their race, religion, background, or disability," he says. "We should help people if they need it, like if they're poor or they can't get around or if it takes them longer to learn something new."

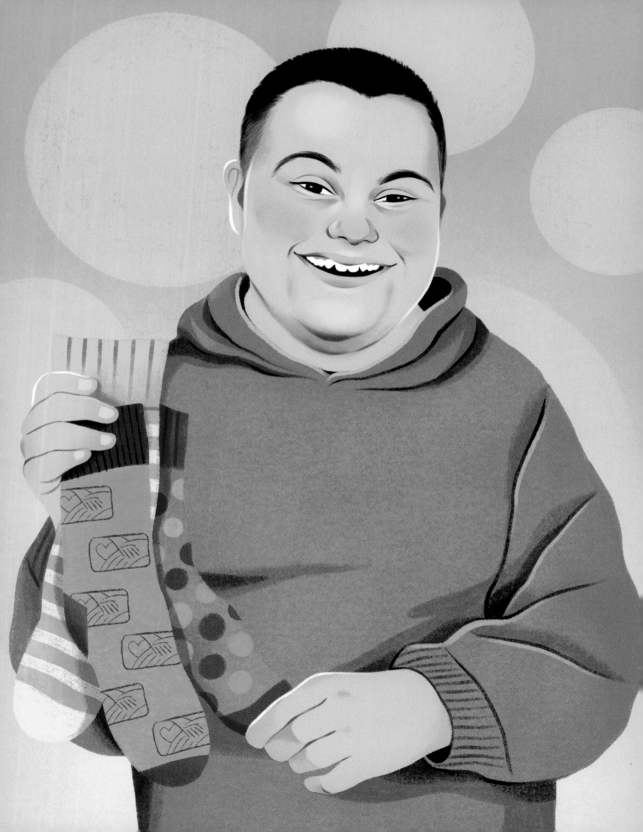

JOHN CRONIN: THE SOCK TYCOON

Home Country: The United States • Born in 1996

Before John Cronin turned one year old, he'd already had two major surgeries—one on his intestines and one on his heart. It took John longer than most kids his age to talk, and he worked for years with a speech therapist. While learning to communicate verbally, he studied sign language and used a device that allowed him to push various buttons with images on them, activating a voice that said phrases like, "I'm hungry" or "I need to use the bathroom."

Back then, no one imagined John would become an international public speaker and the entrepreneur of a multimillion-dollar company. They saw him as a fun-loving kid who liked to dance and wear funny colorful socks.

John grew up in Long Island, New York, with two older brothers and his best friend, José. He and José played soccer together. They had sleepovers and went to Hersheypark for fun. In high school, John took an elective class in fashion, sang in the school chorus, and performed in the school talent show. "My grandfather had just passed from cancer," John explains. "I sang 'Fight Song' by Rachel Platten, and I wore one of his ties as a tribute to him."

John also joined numerous Special Olympics teams, playing soccer, basketball, track and field, and snowshoeing for the organization. He spent weekends training and competing. John wanted to work after school, but he had trouble finding a job because many employers didn't want to hire a person with Down syndrome. (Sadly, only half of teens and adults with Down syndrome have jobs, and many of these jobs are too simple and unchallenging for those with skills in technology and other professions.)

Eventually, John found a job he liked as the mail clerk at a local law firm. He arrived at the office every day after school and ensured that coworkers had enough mail supplies and stamps. He also made the daily run to the post office, sorting envelopes and packages for the fastest delivery. He assisted in general maintenance of the law firm's office, handling the shredding, running errands, and lending a hand whenever he could.

When John wanted something more challenging, he approached his father. "I want to make my own job and work with you," he said. So John and his father thought about what type of business they might start. They remembered his love of colorful socks and decided to open an online sock shop called John's Crazy Socks. They designed a logo and decided on a motto: "Spreading happiness through socks."

Initially, orders came mostly from people around his hometown. Then his neighbors started posting videos of his home delivery on their social media feeds. Suddenly, John and his father could barely keep up with orders coming in from around the country. They literally ran out of socks! At one point, his father had to drive to Kmart stores all over the county to purchase Christmas-themed socks so that John had something to sell on his website.

Now, with the help of his father, John runs a multimillion-dollar company, and John is a sought-after public speaker. One of his favorite memories of public speaking involves the NBA team the New York Knicks. Before one game, the basketball players wore John's Crazy Socks during their warm-up, and before tip-off, John stood calmly holding a microphone in the middle of the court, surrounded by twenty-two thousand fans and basketball players. All the lights went out except for a single spotlight shining down on him. Most other young people would be nervous, but not John. He introduced the Knicks to thunderous applause and cheering from the fans.

In 2019, John became the first person with Down syndrome to win the Ernst and Young Entrepreneur of the Year award, which recognizes the achievements of entrepreneurs around the world. He sells four thousand different types of socks online. Want a pair of pink fuzzy flamingo socks? John's got them. Socks with basketballs, squirrels, or soft-serve ice cream cones? John's got you covered. His own favorite socks are imprinted with pictures of bacon.

John's official title at his company is Chief Happiness Officer, which certainly suits him. With every box of socks he delivers, John still adds a handwritten note, a piece of candy, and a coupon for another pair of socks. He makes thank-you videos, helps to fill orders, and selects the socks for his online store.

During the COVID-19 pandemic, John expanded his role to entertain people around the globe by hosting Tuesday afternoon dance parties on Zoom. In a video clip of one party in June 2020, he spins across the floor of the warehouse wearing bright blue and green socks and a T-shirt printed with the John's Crazy Socks logo. "Socks let me be *me*!" he says.

Every year, he hosts a sock design contest, where anyone from around the world can submit artwork. John turns the winning design into a pair of socks for the winner and offers them a cash prize.

Over half of John's employees have Down syndrome or autism. He and his father donate part of their profits to organizations that support people with developmental and intellectual disabilities. John also works with the National Down Syndrome Society to advocate for job access and fair wages. He and his father have spoken twice to the United Nations—once on World Down Syndrome Day and once at an entrepreneur conference to stress the importance of employing people with intellectual disabilities.

John and his dad appear together on Facebook Live each week for a production they call *The Spreading Happiness Show,* and on the *Spreading Happiness* podcast, they talk about their business, their travels, Special Olympics, and their speaking engagements. "I know things," John says. "I don't just want to lie around. Work makes me happy."

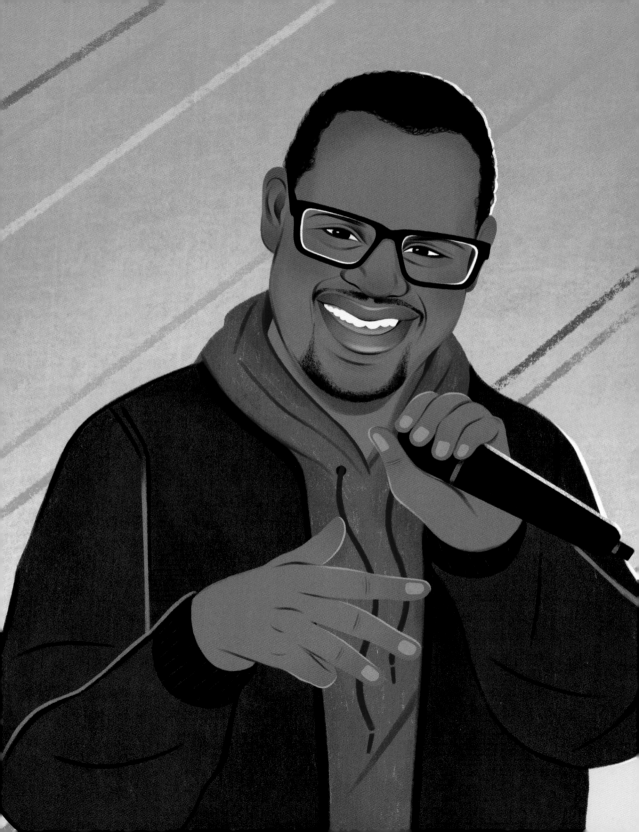

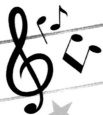

JOHN TUCKER: THE RAPPER

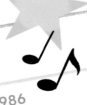

Home Country: The United States • Born in 1986

John Tucker grew up as the baby of the family in Los Angeles with three sisters. He was closest to his sister Trinette; together, they'd sneak out of the house at midnight to go to the market for cookies and muffins. When Trinette learned to beatbox, John sang made-up songs while drumming on the kitchen table. With a love of hip-hop, rap, and R & B, he began to write lyrics about himself, their neighborhood, and their supportive extended family.

John's older sisters were always pestering him to go biking, roller skating, and ice skating. He fell a lot and got discouraged. But music, he says, was a whole different story. "My mom and my sisters didn't know how to rap," he explained. "That was all me." Rapping became John's passion, something he could do well on his own.

In high school, John rapped and danced on the campus quad at lunchtime, surrounded by cheering classmates. Sometimes, he'd get in trouble for making everyone late to their next class. He was a popular, outgoing student, and his classmates nominated him for homecoming king. His oldest sister, Michelle, graduated and went to college, then returned to their high school and became one of his teachers. That turned out to be a great advantage for John.

"If someone tried to tease me, my sister would be right behind me," John says. "Then they'd say, 'My bad, John. I'm sorry, Miss Tucker. I didn't know he was your brother.'"

After he graduated from high school, John joined a theater troupe called Born to Act Players. He began acting in two plays a year while performing all over the city with his dance troupe called Straight Up Abilities. "When I dance," he told Channel 7 news in Los Angeles, "I feel like a superstar." John was living his best life with family and friends, music, and dancing. But then the unthinkable happened—his sister Trinette passed away from kidney failure.

"I became so depressed," John says. "I just wanted to be alone. I locked myself in my room every day and shut my family down. I didn't want to go out."

Eventually John went to therapy. Then he turned to music to help him heal his grief. "I dedicated a song to Trinette," he says. "It's called 'Wherever I Go.'" In one section of the song, he raps, "I can't get you out of my mind. I wish we'd had more time." John misses his sister horribly, but he's found the strength to go on.

Almost a decade later, John's parents heard that the A&E network was planning a reality TV show about young adults with Down syndrome. John's mother called up the producers and asked them to meet her son. He and his family auditioned together over the course of six weeks, and the network finally cast them in the series titled *Born This Way*.

The show, which aired from 2015 to 2019, follows the lives of seven people who meet at a local recreation center. It features their families as well. In the first season, John debuted his first music video, titled "Shake Your Booty," which includes his family and neighbors as background dancers. His friend Jay wrote the beats. In season four, John learns to drive on camera with his costar Steven Clark.

Born This Way established John as a celebrity; the show grew in popularity after it won an Emmy in 2016. Whenever John went to Disney World to perform with his dance troupe, he'd navigate crowds crying, "There's John Tucker!" and demanding his autograph. "I can't complain about that," he jokes. "We will always be an inspiration in the show for other people."

In 2017, John and his *Born This Way* costar Rachel Osterbach became the first people with Down syndrome to present at a major media awards ceremony. They stood at a podium in the Microsoft Theater in downtown Los Angeles during the Creative Arts Emmy Awards, addressing thousands of celebrities. John wasn't nervous. "I've never had a fear of speaking onstage," he says. Nor has he ever had a fear of rapping for strangers. These days, he's working on his new album and getting used to living alone in his Inglewood, California, apartment. He loves to cook eggs, bacon, and pancakes for breakfast and chicken and greens for dinner. "I have to watch my diet," he says. "Sundays are my cheat day. I love strawberry Pop-Tarts."

In 2023, he rapped and danced in *Ride or Die: The Hip-Hop Musical* at the Hollywood Fringe Festival. He also starred in filmmaker Dhar Mann's short film *Passenger SHAMED on Airplane, What Happens Is Shocking* about a man with Down syndrome who sits next to a businessman who bullies him before the pilot and flight attendant step in to put a stop to the man's behavior.

John enjoys attending concerts; he adored getting to see his favorite singer of all time, Missy Elliott, perform live in Las Vegas. "I'm her number one fan," he posted on Instagram in front of a wall of slot machines. In the future, John looks forward to attending more concerts, acting and rapping, and speaking nationwide in support of people with disabilities. "I want people to know that Down syndrome doesn't matter at all," he says. "I'm just a regular person living live to the fullest."

John likes to point out that a lot of kids have Down syndrome or autism, and people should support them with friendship and mentorship instead of ignoring them. He believes in inclusion, where kids learn in classrooms together without being separated. "Don't let disability define kids," he says. "Just keep believing in kids, keep fighting for kids, keep encouraging kids to be who they want to be. Never make a kid feel like he's nothing."

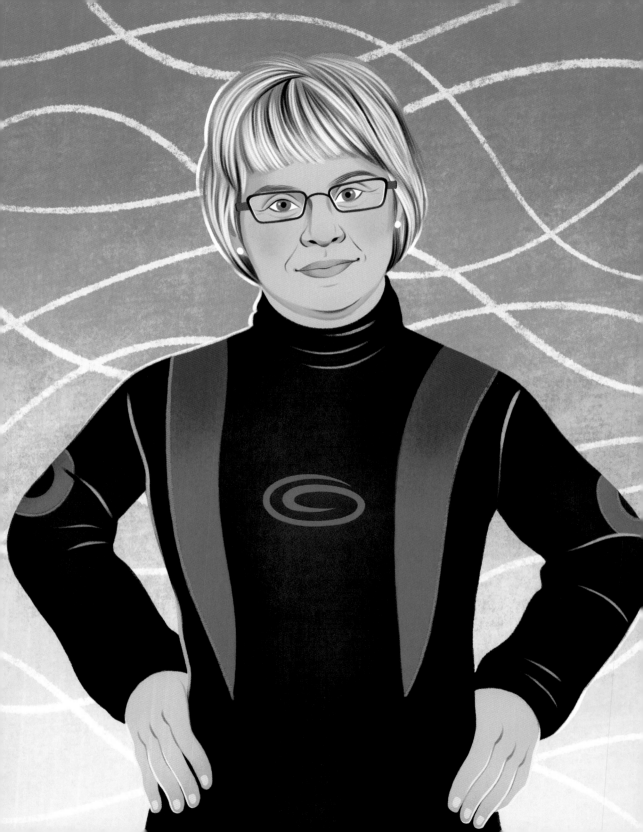

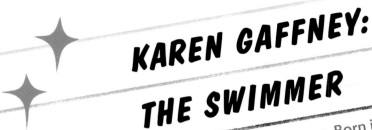

KAREN GAFFNEY: THE SWIMMER

Home Country: The United States • Born in 1977

Karen Gaffney learned to swim before she could walk, when she was only nine months old. When they were kids, she and her brother Brian, who was two years younger, swam laps together at a pool near their house in Portland, Oregon, every Saturday. They'd race each other for M&Ms, which Karen always won...but she shared them with her brother on their way home.

Karen, born with Down syndrome, started an early intervention program when she was three months old. She and her parents worked on activities to help build her muscle tone and fine motor skills. She attended a Montessori preschool for three years before starting the first grade. By the time she began grammar school, she could read, write, and do basic addition! She worked with a tutor twice a week, and her parents helped her preview each week's assignments at home so she would recognize the material at school.

As she was growing up, Karen had to go through several surgeries on her hips. The first one was when she was four years old. Each time that she recovered, she went right back to swimming. When she was seven years old, Karen started in Special Olympics, and she focused on the 25-yard swim—the distance of one wall of the pool to the other.

When Karen was in second grade, another student called her a "retard." She didn't know what that word meant so she asked her parents. That was when they first explained that she had Down syndrome, and it might take her longer than some people to learn things, but she could learn along with everyone else. They told her to ignore the bullies and explained that some kids don't understand what it means to have Down syndrome. They encouraged her to pursue her passions and stay focused on her goals.

As a middle schooler, Karen loved to go to movies, visit her grandparents, and take trips to the beach. In high school, she discovered the plays of William Shakespeare in her English classes. She spent weekend afternoons watching movie versions of plays including

Romeo and Juliet and *The Merchant of Venice* while reading and discussing them with her aunt who was an English major in college.

Karen kept swimming in middle school and high school. She swam for the Catholic Youth Organization in middle school and then for her high school team. Karen received her letterman's jacket her junior year and graduated from high school. Then she earned a degree from the local community college as well as a certificate qualifying her to become a teacher's aide.

In 2001, Karen swam the English Channel—which is twenty-one miles wide—as part of a six-person relay team. Six years later, she swam the width of Lake Tahoe (which is nine miles across) in 59-degree water to raise funds for the National Down Syndrome Congress. The documentary *Crossing Tahoe: A Swimmer's Dream* captured that particular swim in detail: the camera followed Karen in her full wet suit and goggles as she hopped off the boat at 6 a.m. and into the frigid water. For the first forty-five minutes, Karen swam in complete darkness, accompanied by her coach, each wearing glow sticks on their caps so they could see each other

Karen stepped out of the water at the end of the swim to applause from friends and family. She told the film director, "Once people follow my steps and see what I've done swimming-wise, they can do the exact same thing too, if they really put their hearts to it and stick to it."

These days, Karen wakes up at 5:30 a.m., eats a banana, then heads to the pool to swim two miles. After her morning swims, she has breakfast and gets ready for work. Then she goes to work for a law firm in Portland. In her free time, she plays cards with her father, does jigsaw puzzles, and sees Broadway musicals; her favorite is *Wicked*. Karen spends every Friday answering emails for her nonprofit, the Karen Gaffney Foundation, which she founded to support full inclusion for people with intellectual disabilities at home, at school, and in the community.

Often, Karen fields requests for public speaking and travels internationally; she's given talks in Ireland, England, Singapore, Trinidad, and all over the United States. She's particularly passionate about making sure people with Down syndrome are included in clinical trials for Alzheimer's disease. Approximately 40–80 percent of people with Down syndrome develop Alzheimer's-like dementia in their fifties and sixties. Karen herself has lost two friends to the disease. One of them was Lee Jones, a renowned public speaker and self-advocate.

"I think that it's wrong not to study the early onset of Alzheimer's disease in people with Down syndrome," she says. "It's a problem and it needs to be fixed. It is a huge black cloud that hangs over us and our families." Karen makes presentations about this issue in health care settings; she often speaks at Oregon Health and Science University about the capabilities of people with Down syndrome and the benefits of daily exercise and a healthy diet.

Many young adults with Down syndrome and their families grew up listening to Karen's presentations. She's long been a role model for them and for neurotypical kids and adults. Perhaps thinking back to the days when kids made fun of her, she's passionate about inspiring kids to include people with disabilities in their life.

"I want students to understand that we are more like everyone else than we are different," she says. "I know it takes courage to get to know someone who's different than you. It takes courage to invite people to do things with you. It takes courage to get to know more about someone with disabilities."

In the future, Karen plans to give more presentations with the hope of inspiring a new generation to respect and value all people. She plans to continue working at the law firm, a job she loves. And of course, every morning, she'll keep swimming.

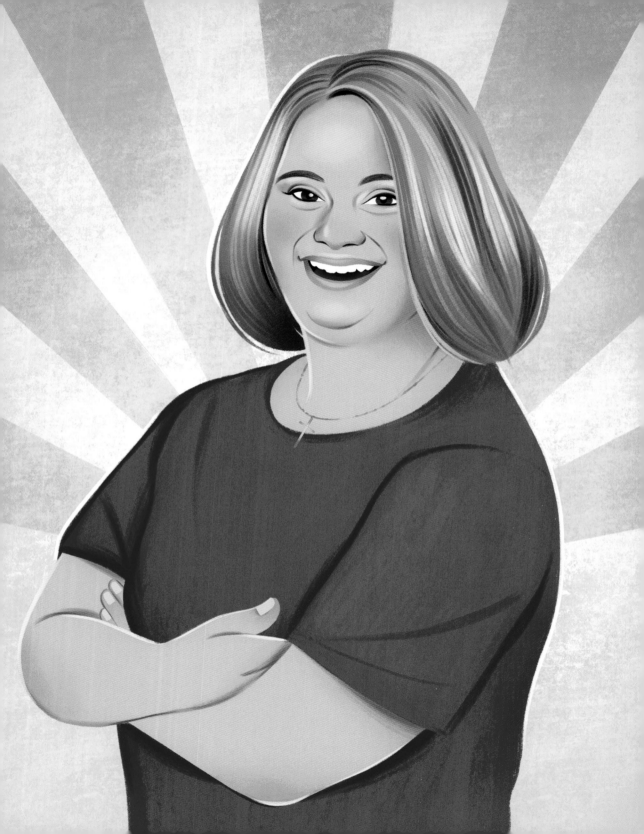

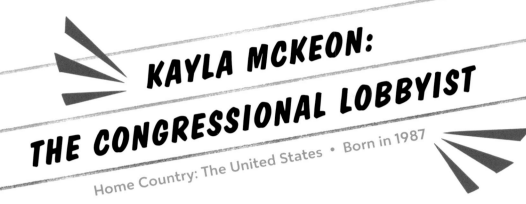

KAYLA MCKEON:
THE CONGRESSIONAL LOBBYIST

Home Country: The United States • Born in 1987

In 2023, Kayla McKeon lifted the top off a sparkling pink box on the *Good Morning America* stage. Before millions of viewers worldwide, she revealed the first Barbie doll modeled after someone with Down syndrome. Kayla, manager of grassroots advocacy for the National Down Syndrome Society, teamed up with the toy company Mattel to make sure the new Barbie looked authentic.

As part of the design team, she suggested the doll have almond-shaped eyes and a straight line across the palm—both characteristics of people with the genetic condition.

"Her dress has butterflies in yellow and blue, which are the colors that symbolize Down syndrome," Kayla explains, adding that Barbie's pink necklace includes three arrows that represent three copies of the twenty-first chromosome, which people with the genetic condition share. "Representation is so important," she says. "Now kids can play with a doll that looks like my friends and me."

Kayla grew up near Syracuse, New York. She learned to read when she was four years old. When she went to elementary school, her parents had to fight for her to stay in regular education classes with her friends. Kayla remembers going to lots of sleepovers as a child. "My friends and I stayed up until three in the morning, just talking and not sleeping," she says. "I loved those sleepovers."

But in the fifth grade, the invitations slowed down, and then they stopped completely. "I have no idea why," Kayla says. "It made me sad." Adding to her sorrow, she found herself in a special education classroom in her school's basement. She sat there miserable and bored, wondering, Why am I not upstairs with everyone else?

In seventh grade, a bunch of students ran down the hall and pushed Kayla into a wall, injuring her. That same year, they teased her until she cried. "That was pretty bad," she says, "but I'm stubborn and resilient. I never retaliated. I have thick skin."

Eventually, Kayla attended regular classes again and found new friends. In high school, she loved English so much that she began volunteering at her local library. After graduation, she attended Onondaga Community College and earned an associate degree in general studies cum laude, which means with honors. Meanwhile, she competed in Special Olympics, playing soccer, floor hockey, track and field, and a unique sport: bocce ball.

In 2011, Kayla got a phone call from one of her coaches. She listened for a moment, then went to find her mother. "I'm going to Athens, Greece!" she exclaimed. She would compete in bocce ball in the Special Olympics World Games. Kayla visited Athens for three weeks, winning silver and bronze medals. "That trip was amazing!" she recalls.

Soon after, her local school district asked her to give a talk to teachers and aides. Wearing an elegant black dress, Kayla stood at the podium with the microphone and spoke to two thousand people about the importance of including people with disabilities in regular education classes. Other organizations began inviting her to speak at fundraising events.

In 2014, Kayla attended a campaign event for John Katko, who was running for Congress. He kept trying to toss Kayla one of his promotional T-shirts, but she never caught one. So after his talk, he walked over, introduced himself, and gave her a T-shirt. A few months later, Kayla attended a charity baseball game, and John Katko was there. She approached him with her business card. It read "Kayla McKeon, Motivational Speaker." "Call me," she told him.

After winning his election, he did give her a call and offered her an internship. In her role, she answered emails and took care of other office duties. Later, Representative Katko invited her to an employment conference with the National Down Syndrome Society in Washington, DC. Kayla jumped at the chance to make her voice heard.

The NDSS president was so impressed with Kayla's public speaking talent that she asked if Kayla would be a lobbyist for the organization. In 2017, she accepted the invitation and moved to Washington, DC, becoming the first registered lobbyist with Down syndrome. Now, Kayla meets regularly with U.S. senators and representatives and asks them to advocate for people with disabilities at both work and home.

"I'm the good kind of lobbyist," she's quick to note. "I'm not the kind that's going to lie and cheat. I'm not like that."

As a spokesperson for the National Down Syndrome Society, Kayla visits Capitol Hill twice a month to speak on behalf of rights for people with disabilities. She believes all people deserve meaningful, stimulating jobs. She's also passionate about overturning legislation that penalizes people with disabilities financially if they choose to get married. "I'd like to marry my boyfriend," she explains. "But he has a disability too, so we would both lose money."

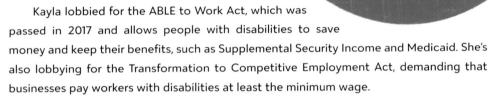

Kayla lobbied for the ABLE to Work Act, which was passed in 2017 and allows people with disabilities to save money and keep their benefits, such as Supplemental Security Income and Medicaid. She's also lobbying for the Transformation to Competitive Employment Act, demanding that businesses pay workers with disabilities at least the minimum wage.

In 2019, PBS produced a documentary titled *My Fight for Inclusion: The Kayla McKeon Story*, which tracks Kayla's life from birth to her current work as a congressional lobbyist. In the documentary, she talks about the Americans with Disabilities Act and how the law needs to better protect the rights of people with disabilities. "I just want to see accessibility everywhere," she says. "We want to be accepted."

When she's not working, Kayla reads a novel a week; she particularly likes James Patterson's thrillers. She loves to knit hats and scarves. "I'm always on the phone," she says. "I'm always talking to someone and asking if they want to go get coffee at Starbucks or Dunkin'." She has a driver's license, and she enjoys getting her nails done and eating at Greek and Mexican restaurants. She lives in her own apartment in Syracuse, New York.

Most importantly, Kayla is thrilled to play a part in furthering the representation of people with Down syndrome in all aspects of life. "We put on our pants one leg at a time," she says. "We are human beings, and we want to be treated like that. I'm just like you."

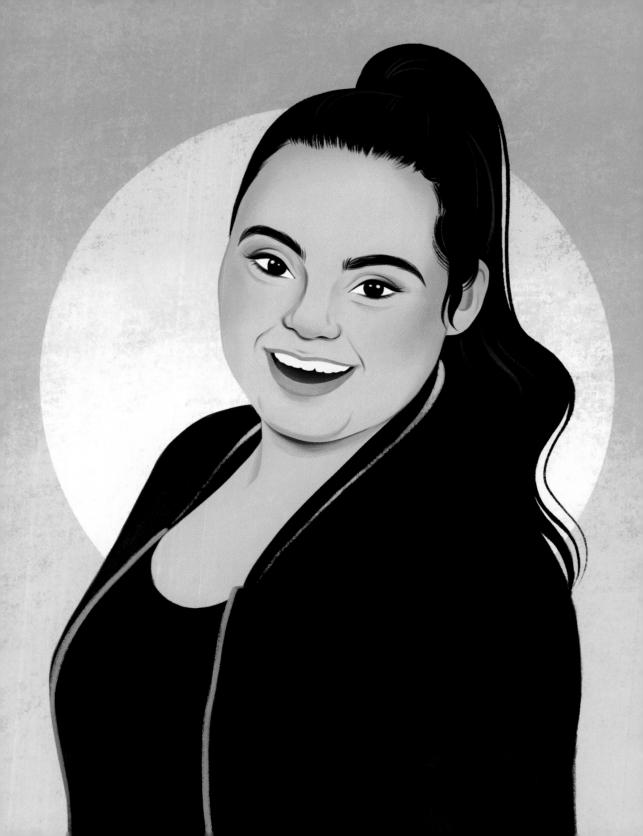

MADISON TEVLIN: THE TALK SHOW HOST

Home Country: Canada • Born in 2001

Madison Tevlin sat across from Chinese-Canadian pop star Tyler Shaw, interviewing him for *Who Do You Think I Am?*, her talk show featuring famous people often judged by the way they look. Tyler began to sing a line from his hit single "House of Cards," and Madison chimed in. "Baby, it's magic, the way you came around," they sang together.

It was a powerful moment for Madison, who'd listened to Tyler's songs over and over as she recovered from heart surgery a few years before. Now, Tyler sat in her studio, talking and laughing with her on camera for all of Canada to see.

"I interview interesting people and get to know who they really are, not judging them at face value," Madison says. "I'm a very curious person. I want people to share their lives, share their story, and I always want people to celebrate themselves and embrace themselves."

Madison is one of the first people with Down syndrome to host a talk show. On her show, she's talked with comedian and actor Ann Pornel who appeared on *The Great Canadian Baking Show*, actor Lane Webber, and drag queen Juice Boxx. When interviewing, Madison doesn't shy away from the hard questions; she and her guests discuss body image, depression, and the pressures of being an influencer. Celebrities open up to Madison, thanks to her outgoing personality and her exuberant laugh.

"My mom always says I'm really witty, and I get people right away," she says. "I feed off other people's energy. For instance, Ann Pornel opened me up more in speaking about what Down syndrome means to me," she says. "We talked about how much fun it is when people underestimate us, and we prove them wrong."

Madison was born in Toronto, Canada, where she has lived her whole life. At thirteen years old, she was a typical teen: she loved hanging out with her sister, Zoie, listening

71

to music, and dancing. She enjoyed singing too—so much that her parents hired a vocal coach in addition to the speech therapist she'd worked with since she was a toddler.

When the coach, Marla Joy, suggested she learn John Legend's song "All of Me," Madison memorized it and decided to record herself singing accompanied by a friend on the piano. Her family posted the video on YouTube for friends to see. A few days later, Madison's video had millions of views.

She was fourteen years old. Suddenly, everyone knew her name. News stations all over Toronto showed the video of her singing, and *Good Morning America* picked it up. Agents and filmmakers started noticing Madison. The next year, she appeared in a Canadian TV series called *Mr. D*. In 2022, she launched her own talk show.

In 2023, Madison earned a Canadian Screen Award nomination for Best Host in a Talk Show or Entertainment Series. She posed on the red carpet in a stunning blue tunic with silver fringe, matching boots, and leggings. Her work and image attracted worldwide attention. When the time came for director Bobby Farrelly to cast his movie *Champions*, he reached out on Instagram to invite Madison to send an audition tape.

Madison just wanted to be a normal high school student, but one of her teachers encouraged her to audition, so she sent in the tape. The director gave her a key role. In the film, which stars Woody Harrelson as a basketball coach for Special Olympians, Madison plays Cosentino, a snarky athlete who helps him learn to respect the skill and value of his team members. "It was so much fun with him," she says. "Every day I walked on set, he'd give me the best hug in the entire world. He pushed me in a good way to become a better actor."

Madison uses her position as a celebrity to work for the rights of people with disabilities. She travels around North America for Best Buddies (see page 112). "It's all about being inclusive and celebrating diversity," she says. In 2023, she attended the New York City Buddy Walk to help raise money for people with Down syndrome. "Not only did I get to go to one of my favorite cities in the world—NYC," she wrote in an Instagram post, "but I got to see my face on a jumbo screen in the heart of Times Square."

When Madison isn't acting or hosting her talk show, she loves to hang out with her mother. "I get a lot from my mom," she says. "My mom got me into fashion," she adds. "I shop basically in her closet. When my friends come over, we're right there trying on her jewelry and all her clothes."

Madison still adores listening to music, in part because she grew up around her Italian grandfather who plays the accordion and the piano. "I've been around music my whole life," she says. "I blast it wherever I go, wherever I am. It helps me stay centered and calm through all my moods and emotions. Just playing it, I feel super good."

Who Do You Think I Am?

Madison describes herself as a foodie with a passion for potatoes. Her family is half Italian and half Russian. "I celebrate all the holidays," she says. "I do all the Shabbat dinners on Friday nights, and we have fun with family and friends who come over and hang out for that." She's particularly fond of December because her family celebrates both Christmas and Hanukkah...and her birthday!

In one of her Instagram photos, Madison models in black leggings and sneakers, a black jacket, and a white T-shirt printed with the phrase she thinks best defines her. It reads "I have Down syndrome and it's the least interesting thing about me."

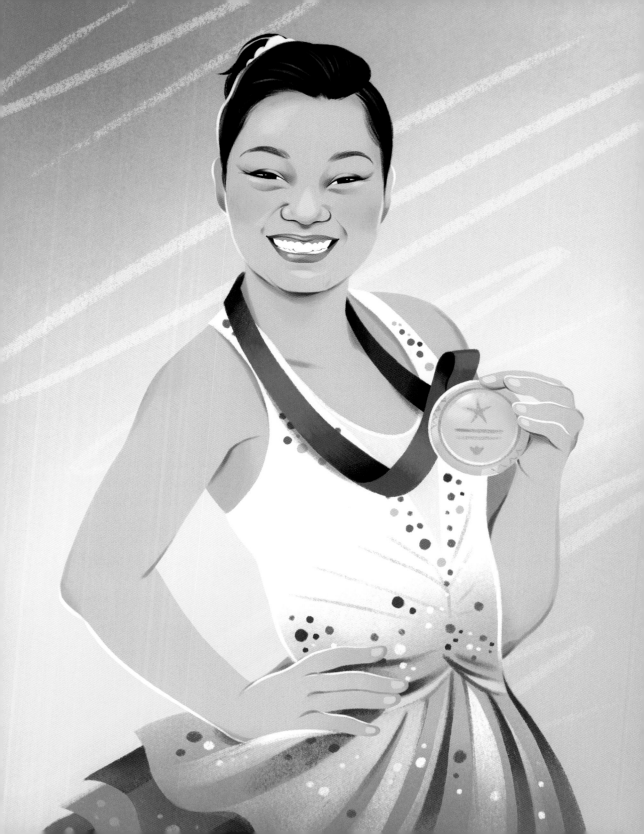

MEG OHSADA: THE FIGURE SKATER

Home Country: Canada • Born in 1994

Meg Ohsada was a happy baby, full of energy, but as she grew older, she became frustrated with her communication difficulties. Speech therapy didn't help very much; she struggled to communicate with words for years. Meg's parents knew she needed a way to express her thoughts and emotions, so they made a decision that would radically change her life.

Meg was born in Toronto, Canada, to parents who had emigrated from Japan, and her young mother was overwhelmed by many unexpected realities. Seeking better personalized medical care for their daughter, Meg's parents decided to move from the big city of Toronto to the small town of Canmore near the Canadian Rockies. The tranquility and beauty of the region helped Meg and her parents to feel calmer.

After her two younger sisters were born, all three girls began to take dance and ice skating lessons. Meg—like others with Down syndrome—had been born with low muscle tone; these lessons helped to build up her muscles while she enjoyed social activities with her grammar school peers. Right away, Meg demonstrated excellent rhythm and balance, and she could memorize complicated choreography quickly. Meg finally found something that helped her express her thoughts and emotions: ice skating and dancing.

Meg practiced at the local ice rink with the Canmore Skating Club, where she trained with former Disney on Ice skater and coach Robin Forsyth. People with and without disabilities got to know Meg at the rink and watched as she grew into an accomplished skater. She also took dance classes in classical ballet, contemporary, lyrical, jazz, musical theater, and hip-hop. Meg joined the Special Olympics figure skating team in Calgary and began to make a name for herself in the sport. At eleven years old, Meg competed in the Special Olympics regional games and won a gold medal. In 2013, at age eighteen, Meg was selected to compete in the Special Olympics World Winter Games in Pyeongchang,

South Korea. With her grandparents watching from the stands, she won two silver medals in figure skating.

The town of Canmore is very small; all the kids attend the same school, and Meg had many friends there. She was shy and quiet, but she found the strength to stand up for any classmates who were bullied by literally standing in between them and the bully.

At Meg's high school's commencement ceremony, teachers awarded her the Danny LeBlanc Memorial Award in recognition of her interpersonal skills, strength of character, and ability to overcome difficulties. All attendees stood up and cheered for her.

After high school graduation, sadly, Meg lost touch with most of her friends. She missed her vibrant social life, but she continued to train in both ice skating and dance. At nineteen years old, Meg had such severe social anxiety that she couldn't talk to people or enjoy what she used to love. Her parents first thought that all the therapies were complete but realized Meg still needed to find a way to express her thoughts and emotions after graduating high school. So Meg started to take medication to help her anxiety and get her back out in the world of athletic competition.

In 2019, she earned two gold medals in figure skating at the Special Olympics Winter Games in Alberta, Canada. That same year, Powerade featured her in their sports drink commercial in celebration of the fiftieth anniversary of Special Olympics. In the commercial, Meg pirouettes in a bright purple skating costume and glides across the rink on one foot. At Special Olympics Alberta's 2020 award night, held virtually because of the COVID-19 pandemic, Meg released a video of herself dancing onstage in a plum-colored dress to the song "Hallelujah." In it, she spins and gestures with the same incredible grace she demonstrates as a figure skater on the ice. "I love expressing myself with beautiful songs," she says.

Meg has more recently taken up rhythmic gymnastics, and she participates in Special Olympics competitions in the sport. In 2021, she was the subject of a documentary film titled *Grace and Grit*, which told the story of how she overcame the low muscle tone particular to people with Down syndrome to become a champion figure skater, dancer, and rhythmic gymnast.

These days, Meg is also an accomplished artist, with her colorful paintings lining the walls of the house she shares with her family. Her portraits and abstract paintings have been displayed and sold in Hong Kong and South Korea. She thinks a lot about the colors and shapes of her emotions. One of her favorite paintings is "Colours of Feelings." In it, she's painted bold strokes of blue, yellow, purple, and pink; she likes it so much, in fact, that it's printed on her business card.

In 2022, Meg met choreographer Daniel Vais, who directs Drag Syndrome, a U.K.-based drag troupe made up of people with Down syndrome. He came to Canada to conduct a dance intensive in which she participated, and he inspired her to think about her disability in a new way. "I feel okay having Down syndrome," she says now. "I have to advocate for myself and my friends." Meg is proud of who she's become as a dancer and figure skater.

She's also proud of her Japanese heritage. In her favorite picture of herself, she's wearing a traditional pink- and white-flowered kimono with her dark hair swept up and accented by a red-ribboned *kanzashi*, or Japanese headpiece. She's rediscovering her history through projects with other Japanese-Canadian artists, and she's planning to connect with artists in Japan. In the future, Meg looks forward to continuing her performances internationally. She's considering moving to her own apartment with a group of her friends.

This year, she and her family watched a touring Broadway production of *Anastasia* in Calgary. She fell in love with the story and asked her coach, Robin, to help her choreograph a routine to the song, "Once Upon a December." Of Robin's choreography, Meg was in awe: "She created drama and magic."

Meg took that drama and magic, and then—after months of training and rehearsals— translated it into a mesmerizing, emotional performance on ice.

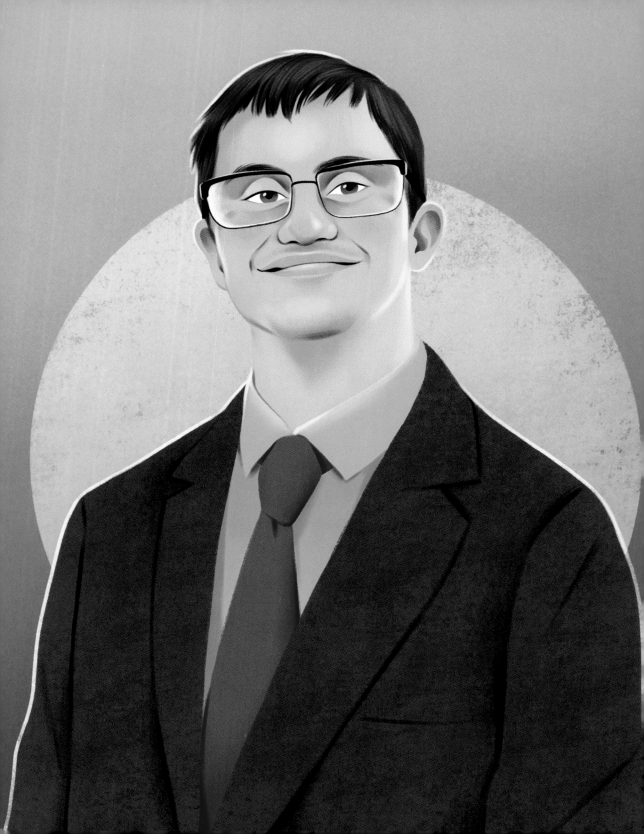

MICHAEL E. HOLTON JR.: THE TEACHER

Home Country: The United States • Born in 1993

In August 2021, Michael E. Holton Jr. was supposed to start a job as a teaching assistant in the technology lab at South Effingham Elementary in Georgia. He was excited because this was the same school where he'd been a student fifteen years before.

And then he got COVID. The illness wiped him out; Michael spent several weeks in the hospital, dangerously sick. But Michael's body was strong and healthy, used to surfing and horseback riding in his free time prior to his illness. People all around his community of Effingham County, Georgia, wrote supportive notes and visited him when he came home. Even Georgia's governor, Brian Kemp, sent Michael a video telling him to keep fighting and wishing him well. Michael eventually recovered and went to work at South Effingham Elementary.

When he was in kindergarten, Michael loved working on computers. His teacher, Mrs. Lee, allowed him to play educational computer games after he finished his classwork. This became a problem when Michael refused to do his work and only wanted to play on the computer. One morning, Mrs. Lee unplugged the computer and told him it was broken. She got busy settling the other kids in to do their classwork, and Michael came up to her. "I fixed the computer," he told her. "It just needed to be plugged in."

Twenty-five years later, he's eager to teach students everything he loves about technology. Each morning, Michael stands outside school in his tan pants, white shirt, suit jacket, and red tie. He greets students as they walk in, sometimes saying hello and other times offering a high five or a fist bump. "I greet the car riders every morning and collect attendance folders from each classroom," he explains. "As a parapro (a paraprofessional, or teacher's assistant), I have huge responsibilities in the classroom with my students."

Michael is the first person with Down syndrome in Georgia to work directly with students in a classroom setting. He teaches 850 students from kindergarten to fifth grade every week. "I love teaching new things," he says. He occasionally teaches fifth grade history lessons and works in the school library. He's coeditor of the yearbook, monitors fifth grade recess, and helps his beloved principal, Mr. Weese, sell sodas on Fridays.

Michael grew up with his parents and his older sister, Jessica. As a teenager, he loved loud music and girls, and he hated cleaning his room. When he was twenty-one, he and his family applied to be on the national TV show *Fix It and Finish It*, and Michael was chosen! The team redid his entire bedroom in a day, turning it from messy and disorganized to tidy and clean, showcasing his surfboard, guitars, and collection of fedora hats.

Michael is also an athletic guy. He studied tae kwon do as a kid, and he was as comfortable on a surfboard as he was on the back of a horse. He's spent many years surfing with an organization called Surfers for Autism, a Florida-based organization that provides free surfing lessons for people with autism and other developmental delays. "It teaches me balance on the board," he says. In 2016, Michael had the chance to meet Bethany Hamilton, the surfer and author who survived a shark attack that left her with one arm. "I have not seen sharks," Michael says with relief.

Michael also participated in equestrian events during Georgia's Special Olympics, regularly bringing home gold medals for his performances on his horse, Slick, who was rumored to love drinking sweet tea.

Michael has always been beloved in his community. In 2012, Michael's high school classmates elected him homecoming king. During the celebratory dance, he danced with the homecoming queen in a shiny burgundy shirt to match his tall crown. After graduation, Michael attended a school-to-work program for people with developmental disabilities. For seven years, he worked at a local hospital in their laundry department. But what he really wanted was to be a teacher like his own kindergarten teacher, Mrs. Lee.

Michael had also been trained as a self-advocate by spending three weekends with other people with intellectual and developmental disabilities. With his newfound knowledge of how to express his needs and desires as well as those of his peers, he first became secretary of the Lowcountry Down Syndrome Society and then vice president. "We all have different abilities, and we all have feelings," he says to his students. "Include Down syndrome classmates in the fun things you do."

Michael plans to become president of the United States someday and fix the inflation problem. He wants members of Congress to better understand Down syndrome and the fact that people with the genetic condition need good jobs and updates to the Americans with Disabilities Act. He keeps up with the latest politics and news, and he loves to learn about history.

For fun, Michael goes to the movies, attends shows at the Savannah Theater, and hangs out with his friends he has kept since elementary school. One of those friends is Kaity White, whom he's known since kindergarten. She now teaches special education, crediting Michael for the inspiration. In 2023, readers of the *Effingham Herald*—the newspaper in Michael's hometown—recognized his passion for teaching. They elected him Most Fab School Support Staff. Watching him high-five students each morning wearing one of his trademark fedoras, jackets, and ties, it's easy to see why.

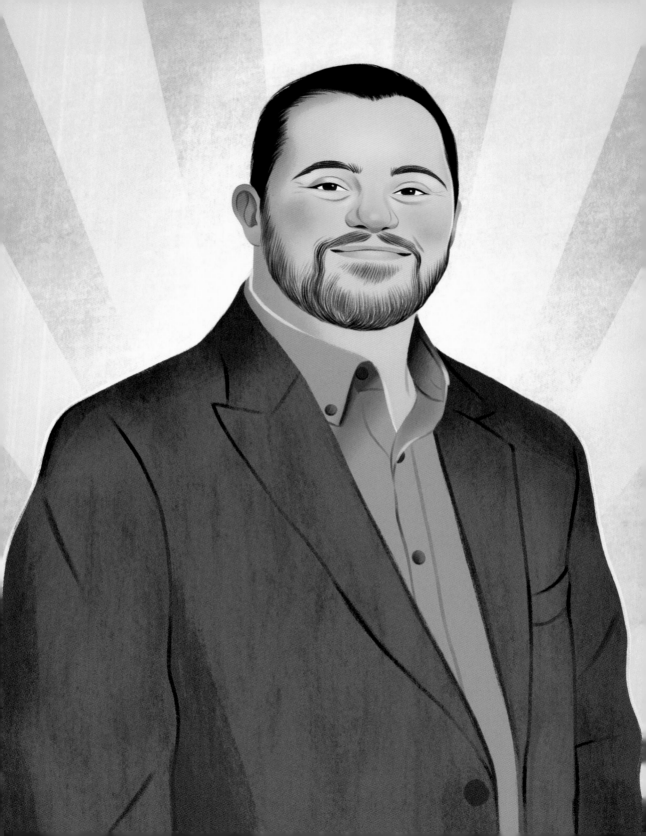

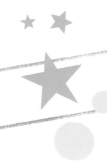

NICK DOYLE: THE COMEDIAN

Home Country: The United States • Born in 1988

Under a spotlight, Nick Doyle sits onstage, pretending to drive an Uber. He's wearing pink high-tops and a matching tie with a crisp white shirt, black pants, and a newsboy cap. One by one, his fellow comedians sit on chairs behind him, pretending to be his passengers. Each is angry; they demand to be taken to Red Lobster. Finally, Nick stomps on an imaginary brake. "We're here!" he yells, and the audience erupts into laughter.

Nick and his costars are the Improvaneers, the first improv troupe made up solely of people with Down syndrome. They entertain audiences all over his home state of Ohio, and sometimes far beyond, with humorous improvised scenes based on games. One of these games is called "Emotional Uber," in which actors ask the audience to provide an emotion (in this case, anger) and a destination (in this case, Red Lobster). They enter the "Uber" with the same emotion but with different reasons for feeling that emotion. The audience finds this hilarious.

"There's also 'Fly on the Wall,'" Nick says about another bit the troupe performs. "Two people sit and talk about a third player, and they don't realize he's there. They talk about funny stuff, and the third player gets annoyed." Nick is usually that third player, inspiring the audience to laugh with his outraged reactions.

"My favorite part of improv is performing for everyone and making them laugh," he says.

Nick studied acting from an early age, performing in community theater productions of *Bugsy Malone* and *The Wiz*. He grew up in a family that has both a great sense of humor and a passion for music and sports. His father is a drummer, and his older brother, Timothy, was a singer and songwriter. Nick began playing the drums at age twelve, memorizing beats to songs by Santana, the Eagles, the Backstreet Boys, and NSYNC, and jamming with his friend Josh, who played the guitar. Nick is so passionate about playing the drums that he has a tattoo of a drum kit on one of his arms.

Nick graduated from high school in 2007. As a young adult, he worked as an assistant coach for the Malone University Pioneers football team. He still loves playing softball, golf, and basketball. "There's no stopping me on defense," he says. He lifts weights to stay strong for all his sports. He's also a good cook; in his white chef's jacket, he's been known to make—in a nod to his Italian heritage—pizza, pasta, and chicken parmesan.

In 2018, tragedy struck his family. His brother, Timothy, passed away from skin cancer. Nick was devastated. Looking for a way to go on, he auditioned for the Improvaneers. The director, Rob Snow, chose him and nine other performers. Nick and his costars trained for a year and a half. They found that studying improv increased their skills in problem-solving, teamwork, and quick thinking. Nick learned about voice projection and eye contact, and his self-confidence and communication skills grew. The Improvaneers' first performance played to over six hundred people in two sold-out shows.

And then the COVID-19 pandemic hit. The Improvaneers had to cancel all their live shows and move them online. In this way, they reached audiences all over the country. Once, they performed with a guest star—improv superstar Colin Mochrie from *Whose Line Is It Anyway?* "I loved it," Nick said. "I absolutely loved it."

Nick's kind and supportive leadership style earned him the nickname "Big Dog." He helped Rob create the Improvaneer Method—a program that teaches improvisational skills to people with developmental and intellectual disabilities. He's the assistant director for both live and online workshops. "Improv builds skills that will greatly increase social and lifetime and workplace opportunities for those with special needs," Nick explains. "We train participants to become professional improvisers and self-advocates."

Nick himself is a professional public speaker and teaches classes on the subject. He tells his students to create a PowerPoint presentation and check that it's working before they go onstage. "Make sure that you move around and engage with the audience," he says. "You've got to have voice projection, eye contact, and, of course, focus. That way, your audience can know about you, and your voice will be heard."

Nick loves teaching, though he admits it can be

frustrating when he's trying to explain the improv games and students talk over him. Still, he perseveres, telling participants to "use what you got so you can say a lot."

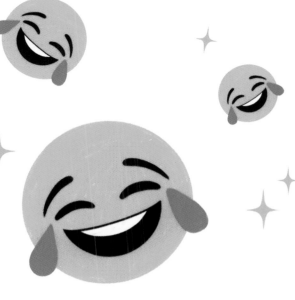

"That means speak up," he says. "Speak from the heart. We have a voice and a seat at the table. We have self-confidence and focus. Having Down syndrome is special, and we're not going to change for no one."

These days, Nick is the vice president of the nonprofit Stand Up for Downs. He's on the board of two nonprofits, and he's just become a Global Ambassador for the National Down Syndrome Society. He's a national sales executive for the Improvaneers, and he travels around the country demonstrating the Improvaneer Method for people. In 2021, his county honored him with the Twenty Under 40! Leadership award.

In his free time, Nick loves to play sports. He watches *Friends* every night with his mom; they even named their cat Phoebe after one of the characters. One night in front of the Improvaneers, he gave a motivational speech to his fellow comedians. "I'm thankful for you guys," he told them. "You guys are like my family. I'm so proud of my castmates, and I'm proud to be a part of this program, and—truth be told—I'm not going to stop."

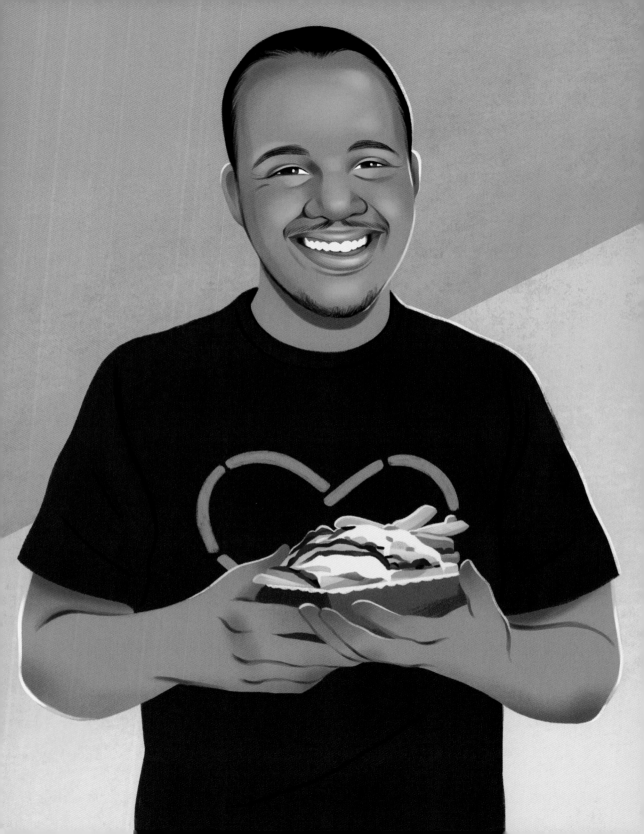

RONNIE BROWN: THE FRY GUY

Home Country: The United States • Born in 2001

When Ronnie Brown was born, doctors inserted a feeding tube into his body because he couldn't digest food properly. He wore that tube for the first six years of his life, and one of the first things he ate when the doctors finally removed it was french fries.

Now Ronnie is a french fry connoisseur and the owner of a business called the Fry Guy. He and his sisters load up a large trailer hitched to the back of their car and set up their tables and portable burners at fairs and festivals around his home near Austin, Texas. On their commute, they sing songs together, such as Flo Rida's "My House."

At the Fry Guy booth, visitors find Ronnie dancing to rap music under a long white banner decorated with a logo of a smiling young man with black hair—a logo Ronnie himself designed. In his booth, it's all french fries, all the time, with specialty toppings that Ronnie created.

With his wide smile, he serves up paper boats of fries with garlic and Parmesan cheese or fries with Texas chili, cheddar, and jalapeños. But his personal favorite is a recipe he invented called the Austin. It's a boat of fries topped with seasoned beef, pico de gallo, queso blanco, avocado, and Guy Sauce. It's a crowd favorite.

"The recipe is a secret," he says about Guy Sauce. "I don't tell anyone."

Ronnie grew up in a big family. He's the youngest of seven kids, with three older brothers and three older sisters. All his siblings looked out for one another when their mother—a former model—became ill with cancer in 2017 and then passed away. "I was sad," he says with tears in his eyes.

School became a place where Ronnie felt safe. He adored his teachers and numerous friends at Hendrickson High School, which is a Special Olympics Unified Champion School. There, the principal and other administrators work with Special Olympics to ensure students with disabilities are fully included in classrooms, sports, student council, and all-school rallies. One of Ronnie's favorite phrases, "I say yes!" even became the Hendrickson High motto. And in 2019, students elected Ronnie homecoming king. For days afterward, he slept in his blue and white crown.

A year later, Ronnie's sister LaTasha and their friend Amber helped him start the Fry Guy. The first day in his new booth didn't go well; Ronnie only sold twelve orders of fries. Soon after, the pandemic hit, so there were very few fairs and festivals for two years. For a while, it looked like Ronnie wasn't going to achieve his dream of launching a french fry catering business.

But Ronnie persisted. He and his family applied for a $25,000 grant from the National Down Syndrome Society and Voya Financial, and they won! Ronnie put the money toward a tent, fryers, and tables. Now, Texas locals and visitors can find the Fry Guy at all sorts of events in the Austin area. Under his white tent, Ronnie takes orders, works the cash register, sauces the fries, and hands customers their food next to a life-size cardboard cutout of himself.

It's Ronnie's job to sample the first batch of french fries for the day to make sure he's serving a quality snack. "My favorite part of my work is being the taste tester," he says. On his website, Ronnie takes catering orders and sells T-shirts, which he models himself. One of his favorites depicts a heart made out of french fries with the words "Fry Love" in the middle.

In the future, Ronnie hopes to own an entire fleet of Fry Guy food trucks and travel to multiple festivals at once. "My face will be on all of the trucks," he says. "And I'll have lots of friends and parties."

Ronnie is a spokesperson and ambassador for the Down Syndrome Foundation of Central Texas. In August 2022, he traveled to New York City to ring the closing bell at the New York Stock Exchange—a privilege reserved for notable businesspeople. He shared this honor with John Cronin of John's Crazy Socks (see page 54), who later featured the Fry Guy on the *Spreading Happiness* podcast.

When he's not working, Ronnie likes to walk around his local lake and listen to Drake. He raps at home constantly and sometimes when he's shopping. He bowls, plays basketball, and runs track and field on Austin's Special Olympics team. Ronnie and his sister Rashida play games of Uno and Thumb War (which Ronnie almost always wins), and she washes and braids his hair every week.

Lately, Ronnie's been working as a model. He walked the runway in an Adidas tracksuit and sneakers during New York Fashion Week in 2021 in a space usually reserved for supermodels. "Those were fresh clothes," he says. "Really nice." His Fashion Week photos ended up on the giant screens in New York City's Times Square for the whole world to see!

Ronnie advocates for the rights of all people to have a fun, meaningful job. Each year, on March 21, Ronnie does a photo shoot in his local park to celebrate World Down Syndrome Day. He hosts a party for friends and family and wears different-colored socks like others around the world who celebrate the awareness day. Often, when he's working, Ronnie wears a T-shirt that reads "Iconic 3," since the number three represents the three copies of the twenty-first chromosome that all people with Down syndrome share. Iconic, to him, means *excellent*. "I want people to see me," he says. "I want them to see my friends with Down syndrome. I want to teach them."

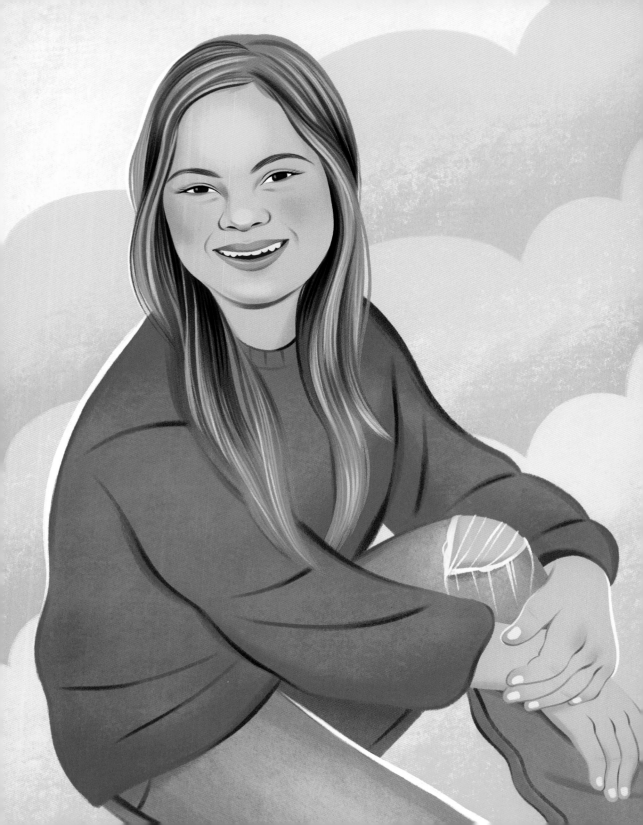

SOFIA SANCHEZ: THE MODEL

Home Countries: Ukraine and The United States • Born in 2009

Sofia Sanchez was born in a small town in Ukraine and was abandoned as an infant. She spent the first fourteen months of her life in an orphanage without parents, siblings, or a home to call her own. Then a man and woman saw her photo on an adoption website and traveled from a small town near Sacramento, California, to Ukraine to adopt her. Suddenly, Sofia had three older brothers, one of whom—Joaquin—had Down syndrome just like her!

"You can make a blended family through adoption," Sofia says. "I love my brothers and my parents and my dogs and my cat."

Six weeks after her adoption, Sofia could use sign language to sign over one hundred words. She loved learning, and she was friendly and outgoing. She began her modeling career at just four years old, appearing in dozens of commercials and print ads for Target. She even did one commercial with her brother Joaquin. Later, she modeled for Hallmark, Abercrombie Kids, Gap, Athleta, and American Girl.

In 2016, Sofia captured worldwide attention thanks to a video her mother posted that went viral. In it, seven-year-old Sofia talks about why people need to stop being afraid of those with Down syndrome. "Yes, I do have Down syndrome," she says to her mother on camera. "No, it's not scary." That video first appeared on *ABC News*'s "America Strong" and then went on to appear all over the world; it's changed attitudes about people with Down syndrome for millions of people.

Sofia and her family have also traveled to Iceland, a country that's made headlines for terminating nearly all fetuses that test positive for Down syndrome. She and her mother work closely with families in Iceland to show them the value of people with this genetic condition. "Down syndrome is not scary," Sofia says. "When you have Down syndrome, it's beautiful inside you."

Sofia is the inspiration for three Scholastic children's picture books, *You Are Enough*, *You Are Loved*, and *You Are Brave*, which she wrote with author Margaret O'Hair. Margaret also wrote *Ride the Wave: Love Sofia and Haole the Surf Dog*. It's the story of how Sofia learned to surf at Santa Cruz Surf Camp with help from a therapy dog named Haole who could ride the waves on a board as well!

In 2023, Sofia attended the world premiere of the movie *Barbie* in Los Angeles, modeling a custom-made blue and yellow dress patterned after the Barbie with Down syndrome that launched earlier that year. Sofia even got to meet and take a selfie with Margot Robbie, who played the title role in the film. "My Barbie dreams come true!" she said in a TikTok video documenting the event.

In her free time, Sofia loves to hang out with her friends by shopping, dancing, and grabbing drinks from Starbucks. "My favorite drink is the dragonfruit Refresher," she says. Sofia also trains and competes in gymnastics and swimming for her Special Olympics region. Her family likes to take vacations, and Sofia's favorite vacation spot is Hawaii's Big Island, where she enjoys water sliding, bodyboarding, and surfing. About the local wildlife, she says, "I love the turtles that ride the waves like in *Moana*."

As a middle-school student, Sofia stood up for kids who were being bullied. "I was a good friend to them, and I gave the best hugs," she says. Whenever she saw other kids sitting alone, she'd walk up to them and say, "Why don't you hang out with me? I'll be your friend." Friendship is also Sofia's favorite part of summer camp. She attends a camp called PALS San Francisco, which offers inclusive weeklong camps for people with and without Down syndrome. "I loved meeting new people and saying hi to everyone," she says. "We went to the Santa Cruz boardwalk and rode the roller coaster."

Sofia has lately broadened her modeling career to include acting and voice-over roles. In *The Hunger Games: The Ballad of Songbirds and Snakes*, she plays Wovey, one of two tributes from District 8. She spent weeks filming with three other kids and a cast of movie stars in Poland and Germany. Sofia also appeared in a short film titled *For Paloma* and voiced an animated character on the Nickelodeon Channel in 2024—the first woman with Down syndrome to do so. She recorded the voice-over on a computer in her parents' walk-in closet with the director on Zoom. "It's funny sometimes, but I like it," Sofia says. "Voice-over is fun. It's acting with my voice. It makes me happy. I could do it all the time."

Sofia started high school in 2023, excited to make more new friends and join the cheerleading team. "We're the Wildcats!" she says proudly. She loves school, and she stays up on current events.

Ever since Russia invaded Ukraine in 2022, Sofia has been deeply concerned about the people in her birth country. "I feel sad about my country having a war," she says. "I don't want them to die. I just want them to have good homes. I want them to have peace and love, away from danger. The world needs to be safe."

Sofia's adoptive parents had to leave several other babies behind when they brought Sofia home. Her mother posted photos and descriptions of them on her blog, and as a result, they all found adoptive families. Sofia herself keeps a picture frame decorated with different-colored buttons in her bedroom. It contains a square photo of her as a baby that her mother took right after she found her. Her big brown eyes stare solemnly into the camera. "I was a cute orphan baby," Sofia says and flashes a big smile. "But I'm not an orphan anymore!"

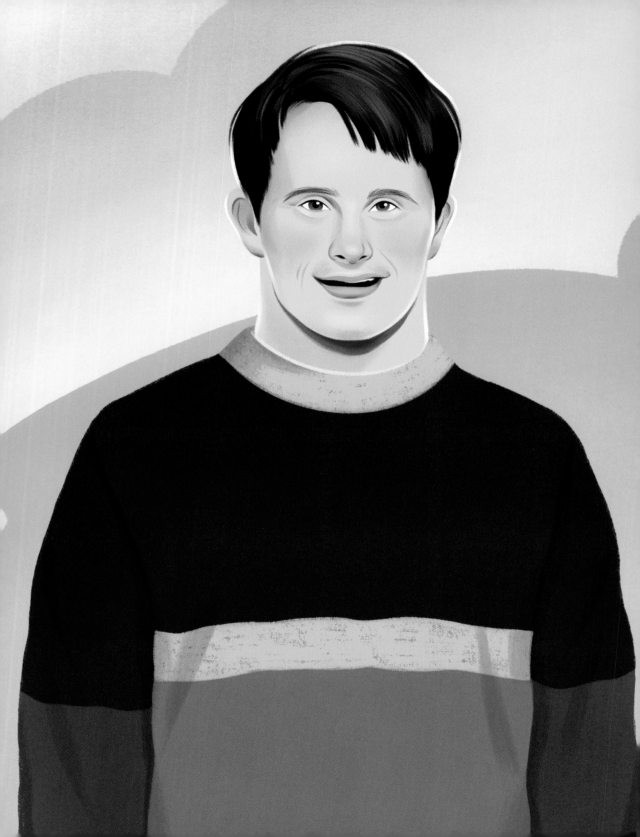

TOMMY JESSOP: THE AUTHOR

Home Country: England • Born in 1985

When Tommy Jessop sat down to write a book about his life, he realized he had plenty of exciting stories. As an actor, he'd played a murder suspect, a teenager who is pushed off a mountaintop, and Shakespeare's famous character, Hamlet. And as a brother, he'd played soccer and cricket and shared jokes with his older brother, Will. The book, titled *A Life Worth Living: Acting, Activism and Everything Else*, recounts Tommy's childhood and young adulthood in Hampshire, England.

He tells the story of waiting three hours to see Queen Elizabeth after a wedding, holding a bouquet of flowers as a gift. Eventually, the queen and her husband, Prince Philip, emerged. The prince spotted Tommy and told him to give the queen the flowers. She was already getting into the back seat of her car, so Tommy hopped in as well. "She was thinking, What is this person doing in my car?" he says. Still, she accepted the flowers with gratitude. Neither imagined that two decades later, Tommy would appear repeatedly in one of her favorite TV shows, the British drama *Line of Duty*.

As a kid, Tommy loved to make people laugh. He enjoyed being the center of attention and being in school plays. He began acting professionally at twenty-two years old and was the first person with Down syndrome to appear in a feature-length BBC movie. Titled *Coming Down the Mountain*, the film follows Ben—a teenager with Down syndrome—and his older brother, who resents the attention, time, and energy their parents spend on Ben. His brother becomes so angry that he tries to push Ben off a mountain, but eventually, he gets to know him and love him. Tommy's accomplishment was all the more impressive because the doctors had told his mother when he was born that he'd never read or talk.

Tommy sometimes speaks with a stutter. He's found that listening to and singing along with rap music help him to speak with confidence. His favorite rappers are will.i.am,

Black Eyed Peas, Nicki Minaj, Eminem, and Snoop Dogg. "Rap has a really fast beat," he says. "It helped."

In his twenties, Tommy appeared in several television shows, including *Holby City*, *Casualty*, *Monroe*, and *Doctors*. He longed to act in live theater, but only a few theaters in England offered roles to people with learning disabilities. So he and his mother founded Blue Apple Theatre, which provides performance opportunities to actors, singers, and dancers with learning disabilities.

At twenty-seven, Tommy became the first professional actor with Down syndrome to play Shakespeare's Hamlet in a theatrical tour around the country. His brother, Will, a professional filmmaker, helped him to understand the character Hamlet's speeches. Will documented the rehearsals and performances in a feature-length BBC documentary titled *Growing Up Down's*, which was nominated for an International Emmy Award for Best Documentary. One of Blue Apple's most powerful plays is *Living without Fear*, which explores bullies who commit hate crimes against those with learning disabilities. Tommy played the victim of a hate crime; he and his five costars performed the play all over England. Police officers, Parliament members and ministers, and hundreds of schoolchildren watched the play. Once, after a performance, a few high school students told Tommy and his mother that they didn't realize people with learning disabilities had feelings and were upset by bullying. Tommy received fan mail from people with learning disabilities who were grateful that someone had finally told their story.

When he was thirty-four, Tommy landed the role of Terry Boyle in *Line of Duty*. He played a man with Down syndrome who was exploited by a gang of criminals and framed for a murder he didn't commit.

In 2021, Tommy and his fellow *Line of Duty* actors attended the National Television Awards to collect their trophy for Best Returning Drama, and the audience cheered and applauded as he broke into a spontaneous dance up onstage. That same year, the University of Winchester awarded Tommy an honorary PhD for his contributions to the arts.

But then the job offers slowed down. Tommy, like other actors with Down syndrome, discovered the lack of opportunities for people with developmental disabilities in film and TV. He spent his time off reading favorite books—especially books by J. K. Rowling and Ian Fleming and biographies of athletes like Spanish tennis player Rafael Nadal—but he longed to work on a creative project again. So he began writing his memoir, with additional sections by his mother, to get his story out into the world and show readers that people with Down syndrome have rich, creative lives. In July 2023, his book was published. He celebrated its release with a party. "We had cakes and champagne," he said. "It was quite wicked," by which he means totally amazing.

In 2023, Tommy and his brother, Will, came up with a fiction story called *Roger the Superhero* and traveled to Hollywood to pitch it to film producers. Along the way, they met *The Peanut Butter Falcon* star Zack Gottsagen (see page 102) and *Scream* star Neve Campbell. Will filmed the adventure and turned it into a documentary titled *Tommy Jessop Goes to Hollywood*, which aired on BBC. "Hollywood is quite wicked," Tommy says.

One producer asked Tommy and Will to send him a screenplay for *Roger the Superhero*, so the brothers got to work writing. You can follow Tommy on his website and on Instagram for updates on the story.

Tommy is a professional speaker, traveling around the UK to campaign for the rights of people with Down syndrome. He was the reporter in the BBC documentary *Will the NHS Care for Me*, in which he investigated the National Health Service and why UK residents with learning disabilities die more often from avoidable causes than neurotypical people.

"We are all different, and we have gifts, skills, and talents," Tommy says. "We just need help to dig them out and to show that we truly are capable. Our lives truly are worth living." He reminds people not to judge a book by its cover. "I actually wrote my memoir to show that life can be exciting for people with Down syndrome," he adds. "I want people to give us more chances to live our lives to the fullest and to be fulfilled."

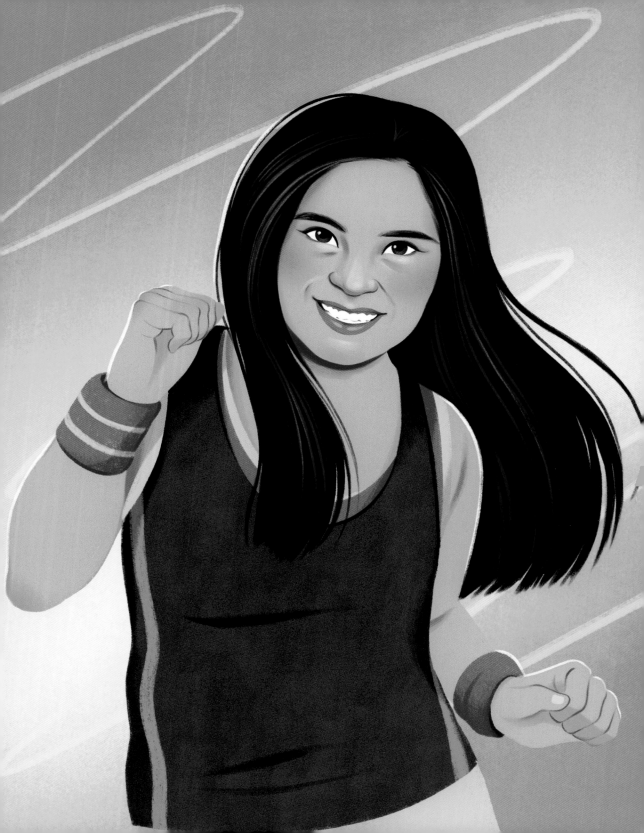

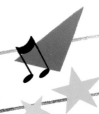

Yulissa Arescurenaga stands at the front of the fitness studio in brightly colored workout clothes, as Havana Brown's "Whatever We Want" thumps from the speakers. She swivels her hips and bounces her shoulders to the beat, with her long brown hair swaying behind her. In front of her, several students copy her movies. They're learning Zumba—a combination of dance and fitness moves—and Yulissa, who was born with Down syndrome, is their teacher.

Yulissa grew up in Lima, Peru. She loved music and dancing to Latin rhythms. She took this love with her when she and her family moved to San Francisco. At ten years old, she entered a local dance contest, and she won! One day, her mother was at the neighborhood gym and heard the familiar beats of Latin music from the workout room. She peeked in and saw people dancing and smiling. When she went home, she suggested to Yulissa that she take the class. At first, Yulissa was reluctant. She thought the gym was all about working out on the machines. Finally, she showed up for a Zumba session. Little did she know that the class would change her life.

Zumba includes a wealth of songs from Latin American singers. Many of the dance moves are inspired by Latin American dances like salsa and merengue. Yulissa adored it all. She told her family that her dream was to become a Zumba instructor, so she began to practice the workout routines, sometimes six hours a day.

Yulissa attended the annual Zumba Instructor Convention in Orlando, Florida, where she was surrounded by other people who adored music and dancing as much as she did. She even got to share the stage with Colombian dancer Beto Peréz. After four years of practicing and training, Yulissa earned her Zumba instructor's license in 2012. She became the first person with Down syndrome to become a certified instructor in the U.S.

One of the reasons Yulissa loves Zumba is that anyone can do it. It feels more like a party than exercise, she explains. "Try it," she says to those who might be worried that people will make fun of them. "People will smile at you."

She teaches Zumba classes at gyms and schools to kids from kindergarten to fifth grade in and around San Francisco, including at workshops for people with physical and intellectual disabilities. She's led the warm-up for several Buddy Walk (see page 120) fundraisers hosted by local Down syndrome nonprofits as well. Yulissa is shy at first when she meets new people, but all her anxiety disappears when she stands in front of a group to teach them the excitement of Zumba!

Yulissa knew her work was helping make an impact when the Alaska chapter of the National Down Syndrome Congress invited her to fly up north to teach for two days. Yulissa, her mother, and her aunt traveled to Anchorage, where Yulissa lit up the stage at Service High School. Wearing lime-green pants and an orange shirt with multicolored bracelets on each wrist, she taught fifty students who were part of the school's partners club, which pairs students with and without intellectual disabilities in sports and other activities. Teachers and students described her as inspiring, amazing, and full of energy.

In 2023, Yulissa taught Zumba in a large ballroom for participants at the National Down Syndrome Congress in Orlando, Florida. While there, she reunited with old friends and posed for selfies with new friends, including Sofia Sanchez (see page 90) and actor Noah Matthews Matofsky, who played the leader of the Lost Boys in the Disney film *Peter Pan & Wendy*.

Yulissa loves to travel, teach, and attend Zumba conferences with instructors from around the world. At home, she likes to watch horror movies, and her favorite cuisine is Peruvian food, especially *pollo a la brasa* (roasted chicken), which she enjoys with salad and french fries. She maintains a collection of five hundred Barbies; each one has a name. Yulissa has had a love for Barbie ever since her grandmother gave her one for Christmas when she was only two years old.

In the future, Yulissa would like to work part-time at Starbucks, but ultimately, her dream is to spread the joy of Zumba to her community. She's recently started teaching for her local parks and recreation department. She hopes people will believe in her work and come dance with her. As she once told the advocacy organization Ruby's Rainbow, "I hope to inspire everyone that with hard work, determination, and pure joy and passion for something, everyone, without exception, can catch their dreams."

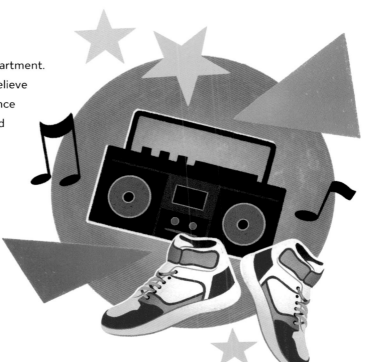

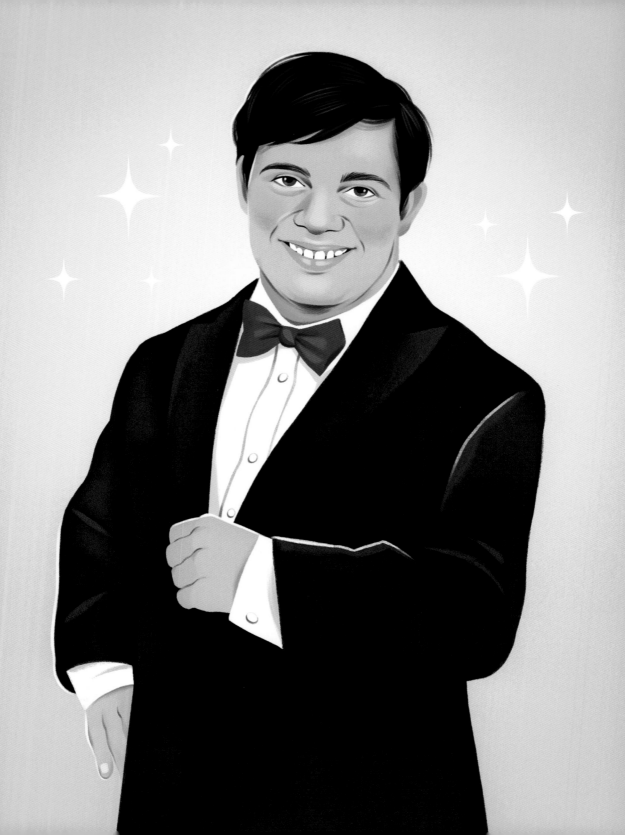

ZACK GOTTSAGEN: THE ACTOR

Home Country: The United States • Born in 1985

Film star Zack Gottsagen stood in a tuxedo next to his *The Peanut Butter Falcon* costar Shia LaBeouf, spotlighted in front of thousands of elegantly dressed actors at the 2020 Academy Awards. Together with LaBeouf, Zack presented the award for Best Live Action Short Film. He made history as the first person with Down syndrome to present an Oscar...a success made even more significant because his mother had to fight for him to be included at school and athletic fields when he was a boy.

Zack grew up in Palm Beach County, Florida, with his mom and younger sister, Elysha. At age three, he portrayed a frog in a preschool play, and he knew right then that he wanted to be an actor. But Zack would travel a long, difficult road to make that dream a reality.

Zack experienced a great deal of discrimination as a child. In first grade, he joined a Little League baseball team with his friends, but the coaches kicked him off the team after the third game when they realized he had Down syndrome. Fortunately, the Americans with Disabilities Act was signed into law in 1990, when Zack was five years old, to increase the civil rights of people with all disabilities.

So when the coaches told Zack's mother that he could no longer play on the Little League team, she had the ACLU threaten to file a lawsuit, which became one of the first disability discrimination cases in the country. The ACLU demanded that every Little League coach and assistant coach in the United States be trained on how to include kids with all disabilities on their teams. Zack's family won the case, and he finished the season with his friends as both a second baseman and a catcher.

Still, Zack struggled for respect and understanding in school. When he was six years old, educators refused to teach him how to read. They believed he wasn't capable of it. But Zack knew that as an actor, he would have to read movie scripts, so his mother hired a tutor to teach him to read after school. As he moved through elementary school, he made many friends.

Sadly, when Zack graduated from fifth grade, he encountered further discrimination in the middle school he was supposed to attend. Staff at the school refused to let kids with disabilities eat lunch in the cafeteria with their nondisabled peers. Zack was devastated, but it didn't destroy him. Encouraged by his mom and educators from his elementary school, he applied for Bak Middle School of the Arts and was accepted. He loved getting to study acting.

At the end of eighth grade, Zack was eager to continue his studies in acting, so he auditioned for Dreyfoos School of the Arts. The first time, educators rejected his application. His mother, having watched the way teachers and coaches had treated him over the years, filed a complaint with the Office for Civil Rights in the Department of Education. The office did an investigation and found that the Dreyfoos School of the Arts had never accepted a student with a disability.

Zack and his mom argued that people with disabilities have artistic talents that have nothing to do with Down syndrome, autism, etc. The U.S. Department of Education's Office for Civil Rights required the school to reaudition him and others with disabilities or close the school. This time, he was accepted.

In high school, Zack met a classmate named Adam Sussman; they became friends and formed an activity club called Bring Kids Together, which was made up of people with and without disabilities who just wanted to hang out and have fun. Students from all over the school district joined the club. Zack and Adam—who now works in reality television—have stayed friends for decades.

Zack graduated from high school as a theater major with a dance minor and took classes at Palm Beach State College. In his twenties, he worked as a dance and theater teacher and at his local movie cinema. He attended film camps with Zeno Mountain Farm in Venice, California, and appeared in several short films, including *Bulletproof*. After that, Zack suggested to his screenwriting friends Tyler Nilson and Michael Schwartz that they write a movie where he was the lead actor.

The result was *The Peanut Butter Falcon*, one of the first feature-length films to have a main actor with Down syndrome. This film became the number one independent film in 2019. Also starring LaBeouf and Dakota Johnson, it's an adventure story about a young man named Zak who has Down syndrome and runs away from a nursing home to pursue his dream of becoming a professional wrestler.

In the film, Zack captivates audiences with his comic delivery of lines like, "You are not invited to my birthday party!" He does all his own stunts, shimmying between the bars on a window, turning a backward somersault onto the lawn, and plummeting thirty feet into a lake. His favorite scene from the film is when he dances with Dakota Johnson beside a campfire. "I still remember that night," he says.

After *The Peanut Butter Falcon*, Zack appeared in the films *At Last* (with George Lopez), and *God Save the Queens*. He also starred as a mail carrier in a music video titled "What's Done Is Done," produced by the rock band Delta Spirit and costarring Jamie Brewer (see page 46).

Zack has lived in an apartment near his mother since he was twenty-one years old. "I am a very nice person," he says. "I'm funny and very cool, and I am a good role model. People always come to me for advice." When he's not acting, Zack loves to go to parties and hang out with his family, friends, and his rescue dogs. He also plays basketball, swims, runs, bowls, and goes to movies.

In 2023, he appeared in a play titled *label*less* in Cincinnati, Ohio. In it, he wrote and performed a spoken-word poem that begins, "Look at me. What do you see? My disability? That is not me. Look harder. See my talent. I have a dream. Just like you."

EVENTS AND GROUPS

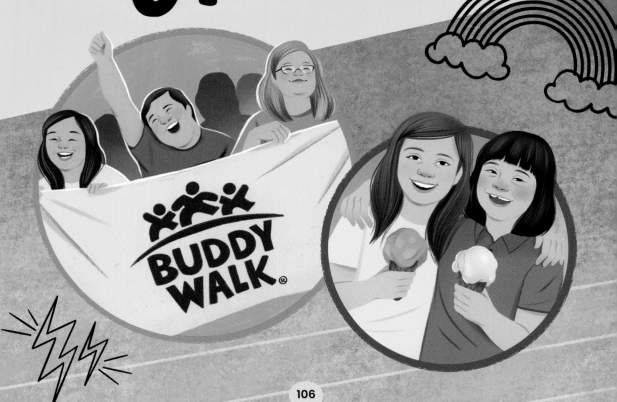

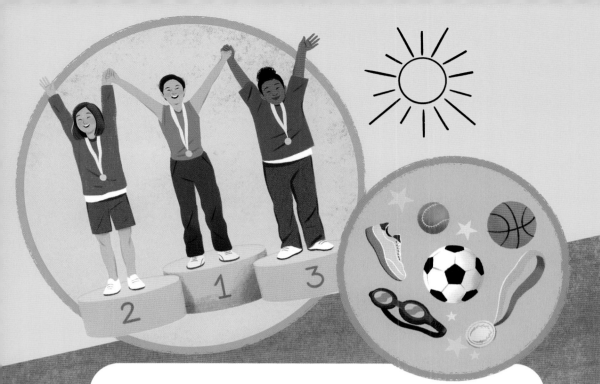

ACROSS THE COUNTRY and around the world, many organizations exist to serve children and adults with Down syndrome and their families. Some focus on helping people with intellectual and developmental disabilities (IDD) to achieve their athletic goals. Others offer resources ranging from healthcare to political activism. Some groups help people with Down syndrome to find their perfect jobs and living situations. Others provide physical and virtual spaces for people to simply hang out, talk, and have fun.

Each of the groups in this book has a governing board that includes people with Down syndrome who lend their time and insights to make sure the rights of people with IDD are respected. Each group relies on volunteers to do everything from helping out at athletic events and fundraising benefits to becoming a good friend to someone with Down syndrome. Read on, and you just may find yourself signing up to volunteer with one of these organizations!

SPECIAL OLYMPICS

What if you loved watching baseball and basketball, track and field, swimming, or figure skating on TV, but you never got a chance to try these sports yourself? This was the situation for many people with Down syndrome before 1962. Doctors, coaches, and parents didn't believe they could learn to play sports, much less compete in them.

But then Eunice Kennedy Shriver—one of President John F. Kennedy's sisters—heard about a woman unable to find a summer camp for her child who had an intellectual disability. The challenge resonated deeply with Eunice because her sister Rosemary was born with an intellectual disability as well.

So Eunice decided to start a summer camp for children with disabilities at her farm in suburban Washington, DC. Thirty-four children and almost as many counselors were invited to swim, play basketball and soccer, and ride horses. Eunice ran Camp Shriver for four years. Eventually, people from the public school system and the parks department took notice of how much fun the kids were having. They loved watching the friendships that blossomed between neurodiverse and neurotypical children; Eunice's own son Tim swam, ran, and played with a boy his age who had an intellectual disability.

Camp Shriver inspired Special Olympics, an organization that helps people with IDD to develop their athletic and social skills through year-round sports and competition. More than that, Eunice and her brother Senator Edward Kennedy were leaders of the Joseph P. Kennedy Jr. Foundation. Together with the Chicago Park District, the foundation planned and paid for a daylong sports competition serving people with IDD, modeled after the Olympic Games.

In July 1968, a thousand athletes from Canada and the

United States gathered at Chicago's Soldier Field to watch a teenage athlete bearing a torch in one hand as he ran up to the forty-five-foot-tall John F. Kennedy Flame of Hope. He lit the fire, signifying a new era for people who'd previously been hidden away in the shadows.

Organizers released two thousand balloons into the sky, and Eunice took the stage to speak the famous words that would become the Special Olympics oath: "Let me win," she said. "But if I cannot win, let me be brave in the attempt."

That first year, athletes competed in over two hundred events, from water polo and floor hockey to sprinting and swimming. Scientists at the time believed that swimming was too dangerous for athletes with IDD, so Special Olympics recruited numerous Red Cross volunteers to stand by. As swimmers participated in the twenty-five-yard freestyle and backstroke, lifeguards stood alongside the pool in case of emergencies. But there were no emergencies, and at the end of the day, each winning athlete went home with a gold, silver, or bronze medal. The first Special Olympics competition proved so successful that Shriver and the others agreed to hold the event every two years.

Later that year, Senator Edward Kennedy made Special Olympics an official

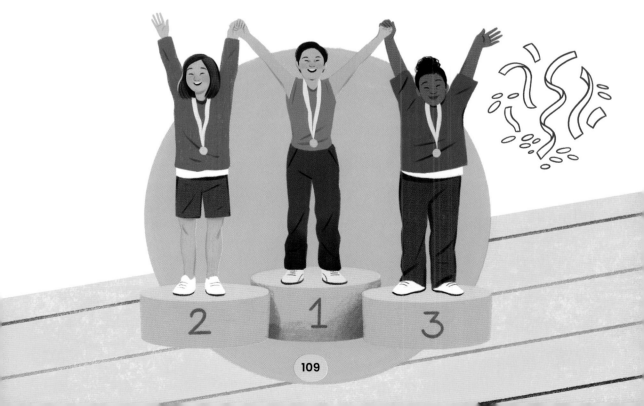

organization. Since then, the organization has grown to include over six million athletes and a million coaches and volunteers all over the world. Participants can choose from more than thirty sports including snowboarding, gymnastics, figure skating, and powerlifting. Regions around the world hold their own practices and competitions, and the organization sponsors over one hundred thousand competitions each year!

The Special Olympics World Games has taken place all over the world, including in Berlin, Dublin, Abu Dhabi, and the home of the first modern Olympics: Athens, Greece. Many celebrities have spoken over the years about the importance of Special Olympics. In the 1970s, Bob Hope and Frank Sinatra supported the organization. Recently, actor-director Lin-Manuel Miranda, NBA all-star Andre Drummond, and singer-songwriter Avril Lavigne have voiced their support for Special Olympics.

Special Olympics athletes with Down syndrome have set impressive records. In 2016, golfer Amy Bockerstette became the first person with the condition to receive an athletic scholarship from a college and compete in a national collegiate championship. In 2020, Chris Nikic (see page 22) became the first Special Olympian with Down syndrome to compete in a full Ironman race, swimming 2.4 miles, bicycling 112 miles, and running 26.2 miles as part of the competition.

In 2021, Abigail Adams became the first woman with Down syndrome to complete a sanctioned sprint triathlon—a half-mile swim, 3.1-mile run, and 10.6-mile bike ride. Like Chris, Abigail and her boyfriend, Chad, train with Florida's Special Olympics team and compete together around the U.S.

In 2022, Abigail competed in the triathlon and appeared as the keynote speaker during the opening of the Special Olympics USA Summer Games. She strode up to the podium in a red shirt and matching red sneakers. "When you refuse to give up, you send a message to every village, every city, every nation. A message of hope, a message of victory!" she said to cheering crowds in the stands. Then she pumped her fist, flashed a bright smile, and cried, "Never give up!"

Anyone can volunteer in support of Special Olympics. The organization welcomes assistance in coaching, fundraising for uniforms and travel expenses, cheering in the stands during competitions, and more. Kids ages fourteen and under are welcome to volunteer if they're accompanied by a parent or caregiver.

The organization oversees fun and creative annual fundraisers. In the Polar Plunge, held around the world each winter, participants ask for financial donations from friends, family, and community members before they jump into an icy lake, river, or ocean! In the Plane Pull, teams raise money for the privilege of competing against one another to see which group can pull an airplane with a rope across the tarmac the fastest.

Many of the people profiled in this book speak of Special Olympics as the reason they have a community of friends as well as the reason they stay in peak performance shape and achieve their dreams. The organization has inspired Abigail to train for an Olympic triathlon—double the distance of her sprint triathlon.

"You've got to stay true to who you are, believe in yourself, and have motivation!" she says. Special Olympics helps athletes from around the world do just that while improving their physical fitness in the midst of an exuberant athletic community.

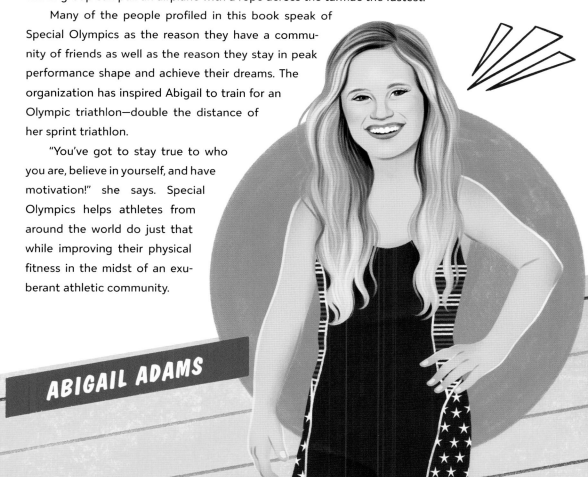

ABIGAIL ADAMS

BEST BUDDIES INTERNATIONAL

Imagine eating lunch alone in the cafeteria and then watching your classmates head off to one another's houses for after-school playdates and weekend birthday parties without getting an invite yourself. Watching others participate in things you're excluded from can feel isolating. Volunteers at the nonprofit Best Buddies International want to make sure no one with IDD feels isolated.

Launched in 1989 by Anthony K. Shriver, the son of Eunice Shriver, Best Buddies creates friendships between people with and without IDD. Respect and kindness are core values of Best Buddies. The organization also helps people find jobs and apartments, enabling them to live fulfilling independent lives. Endurance swimmer Karen Gaffney (see page 62) serves on the Best Buddies advisory board, raising money and awareness for the program.

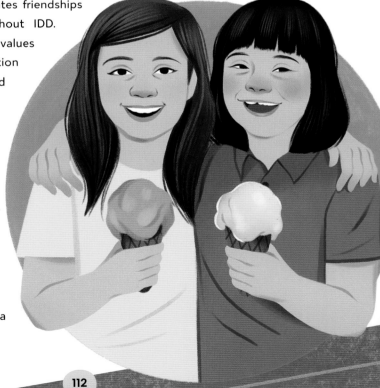

"We want to have friends," she says of people with Down syndrome and other IDD. "We want to be included in every-thing." Speaking from a podium at a

Best Buddies conference, she told a cheering crowd, "You all have the ability to be a friend to those around you even if they seem different than you."

The Global Ambassador program provides training for people with and without IDD, teaching them how to write and deliver speeches and advocate for themselves and the rights of others. Football quarterback Tom Brady is a Global Ambassador, as are actor and influencer Olivia Culpo, NBA all-star player Al Horford, and celebrity chef Guy Fieri. Lauren Potter, who played the character Becky Jackson in *Glee*, is a Global Ambassador as well. She's worked with Best Buddies and Special Olympics on their antibullying campaign called Spread the Word to End the Word. She starred in a public service announcement with *Glee* costar Jane Lynch too. "It is not acceptable to call me a retard," she says in the PSA, "or call yourself or your friends retarded when they do something foolish."

Middle-school and high-school students can sign up for the Best Buddies program. Those with IDD get matched with neurotypical kids their same age. Buddies do a variety of fun activities together, from going to movies and bowling, to dancing and watching sporting events. College students can sign up as well, and there's even a remote Best Buddies option for people who are more comfortable getting to know one another at home on their computer.

Canadian actor and talk show host Madison Tevlin (see page 70) says getting matched up with a friend through Best Buddies meant everything to her as a kid. At a conference near her home in Toronto, she stood in the Best Buddies signature purple T-shirt and talked about how the organization contributed to her becoming happier and more confident. "Making new friends hasn't always been easy for me," she told the audience. "The added pressure of

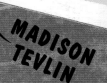

MADISON TEVLIN

starting high school and being a teenager seemed to make everything worse. All of this left me feeling really isolated and alone."

When she joined the program, Madison was matched with a student named Sierra. They went to school dances and Blue Jays games, bowled together, hung out at each other's houses, and attended each other's birthday parties.

Now Madison works as a Global Ambassador for Best Buddies.

AC Heigl (see page 18) is also a longtime participant. She belonged to the Best Buddies friendship club at her Indiana high school; her buddy was Maria Schultz. Together, they got manicures, went out to dinner, made cookies, and sang Taylor Swift songs. In September 2022, AC moved into the organization's Georgetown apartment with a friend from her university plus two neurotypical roommates. She loves how the Best Buddies community has become her family. She and her housemates enjoy playing Jenga, working out, and watching *The Bachelor* together.

The organization has a vibrant Instagram feed with over one hundred thousand followers. Visit it, and you'll see pictures of smiling friends brought together by the organization. In California, Brian and Josue met at a Best Buddies bowling party and bonded over a love of soccer; they've gone out dancing, to a painting party, and to each other's houses to hang out. Another friendship pair—Maggie and Aidan from Ohio—explain on Instagram that they bowl, watch movies, and go on shopping trips together. Aidan, who is neurotypical, now wants to become a special education teacher thanks to her friendship with Maggie.

AC HEIGL

Best Buddies participants with IDD often explain in social media posts that they no longer feel lonely and isolated thanks to their buddy. Some neurotypical participants eventually work for Best Buddies, inspired by the relationships they've created in the program.

Does your school have a chapter of Best Buddies? If not, you can start one. With the help of a teacher or other adult leader, you can identify kids with and without IDD who want to be part of a friendship club. Register your club online, and let the fun begin!

NATIONAL DOWN SYNDROME SOCIETY

I n 1978, a young woman named Betsy Goodwin gave birth to a beautiful baby girl named Carson. But then the doctor said something that chilled Betsy and her husband, Bart, to the bone. "Your baby has Down syndrome," he told them. "You shouldn't bring her home."

In the 1970s, doctors had very little information on people with this genetic condition. Many believed that parents should place their children with Down syndrome in an institution without access to school, athletics, arts, or the outdoors. The idea of giving up their baby broke the Goodwins' hearts.

Instead, they brought Carson home. And then they got to work educating themselves and sharing any information they could find about how to help children with Down syndrome thrive. The result of their research and efforts became the National Down Syndrome Society (NDSS), the human rights organization that Betsy launched in 1979 with her friend, Dr. Arden Moulten.

Decades later, NDSS is teaching everyone—from medical professionals to teachers to coaches to students—how to include people with Down syndrome in all aspects of life.

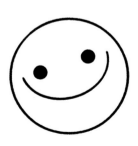

Charlotte Woodward is the education program associate for NDSS. She was born with Down syndrome and earned her sociology degree from George Mason University with a concentration in inequality and social change. "People with Down syndrome should be at the table when decisions are being made about their lives," she says.

Charlotte assists her coworkers at NDSS with multiple projects. One of these is the Buddy Walk, a mile-long walk that raises money for research and programs beneficial to people with Down syndrome. In 1995,

Chris Burke led the first Buddy Walk in New York City. Chris was the first actor with Down syndrome to appear as a main character in a prime-time TV show, titled *Life Goes On*. Now, people with Down syndrome and their families and friends participate in the Buddy Walk in cities around the world. Each year, the event raises millions of dollars.

"We put on charity races, and we have an ambassador program to teach and empower people to advocate for themselves on a systemic level," Charlotte says. "We also have a wonderful education program where we fight for the rights of people with Down syndrome to access free and appropriate education at school."

The NDSS website provides a wealth of resources for employment, health, and wellness, and people have access to individual chapters around the country. The organization also hosts the annual Down Syndrome Advocacy Conference in Washington, DC, for over a hundred people with Down syndrome from the U.S. The advocates dress in business suits and spend a day talking with U.S. senators and congresspeople about issues that affect them, including the law that financially penalizes people with disabilities if they get married and the lack of meaningful jobs and fair pay for people with IDD.

Charlotte Woodward is particularly passionate about making sure people with Down syndrome don't sit at home day after day, lonely and bored. "I always say that exclusion and seclusion do not equal inclusion," she says. "Being employed at NDSS has given me a sense of inclusion and belonging as well as a sense of community. The more inclusion and belonging you can find in integrated employment spaces, the more opportunities you have

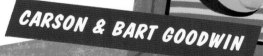

CARSON & BART GOODWIN

access to," she explains. "And the more opportunities you have access to, the more accomplishments you'll have."

Many members of NDSS with Down syndrome talk about their accomplishments on TikTok, Instagram, and Facebook, describing their work, their passions, and their frustrations.

Charlotte is a tireless advocate for the rights of people with Down syndrome, whether she's working from her home in Fairfax, Virginia, or advocating to members of Congress on Capitol Hill. She's on a first-name basis with many U.S. representatives and senators.

Born with a congenital heart defect, Charlotte was one of the first people with Down syndrome to receive a heart transplant. During the process, she learned that many surgeons worry about doing an organ transplant on people with the genetic condition, questioning their worthiness to receive a transplant and their ability to adhere to posttransplant protocol and care. To fight against this way of thinking, Charlotte and NDSS worked with Senators Marco Rubio and Maggie Hassan to write a bill. "We have inherent value and worth," Charlotte says. "We deserve more."

So much has changed since Betsy and Bart Goodwin decided to bring their baby daughter home instead of putting her in an institution. Thanks to their original vision and dedication, NDSS has spent decades making sure people with Down syndrome get a seat at the table and an opportunity to weigh in on everything from homelife and employment to marriage and who gets an organ transplant.

Anyone can get involved with the NDSS. You can sign up on their website to help with a Buddy Walk in your area or participate in Racing for 3.21—an annual event that asks people to walk, run, bike, hike, or swim to raise money for the work that NDSS does. You can write to your congresspeople in support of legislative changes to improve the lives of people with Down syndrome. You can share NDSS's social media posts to increase public awareness of their programs and participants.

"We want people to look beyond our disability diagnosis and see us for who we are as individuals and people with dreams, wants, and desires," Charlotte says. "Having a disability is a natural part of life, and it's very important to have friends and employers who can give you a sense of inclusion and belonging." Her words sum up the values of all who belong to the NDSS.

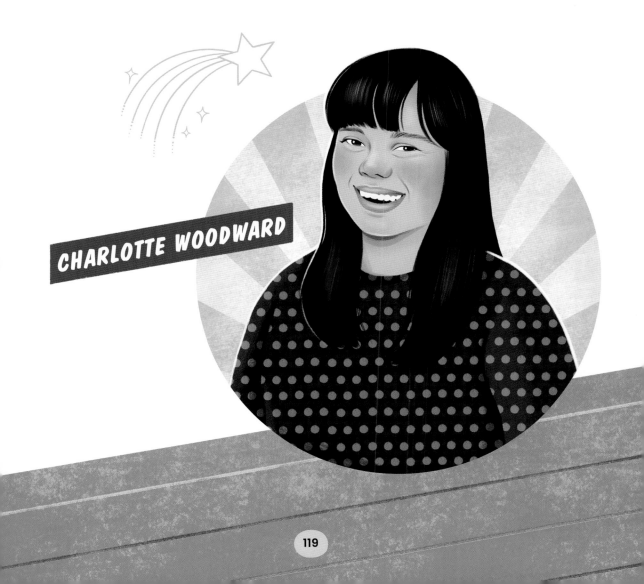

CHARLOTTE WOODWARD

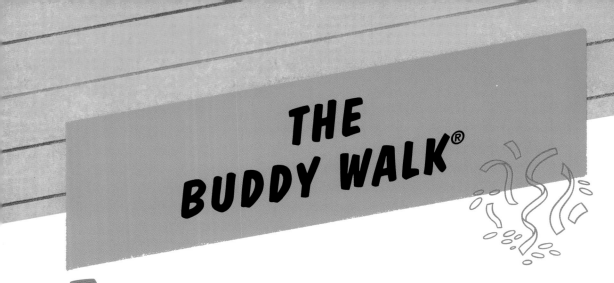

THE BUDDY WALK®

The Buddy Walk® is an enormous party happening all around the world—usually in the fall—to raise awareness of people with Down syndrome and raise money for the nonprofits serving kids and adults with the genetic condition. Think live music and dancing in the streets! Think costumed characters like Batman and Barbie giving high fives and posing for photographs. During the Buddy Walk, people with Down syndrome, along with their friends and families, walk or run a mile. They're joined by firefighters, police officers, schools, scouting troops, cheerleaders, college sororities and fraternities, and anyone else who wants to come out and cheer for diversity and inclusion. Sometimes, even well-behaved dogs attend!

The National Down Syndrome Society (see page 116) launched its first Buddy Walk in October 1995. Families and kids with Down syndrome traveled to New York City from fourteen different states to show the world what they could do. Kids gazed up at photos of themselves, larger-than-life on the iconic jumbotron screen in Times Square. And then *Life Goes On* star Chris Burke gave an inspiring speech and led people on a one-mile walk through Central Park.

That inaugural year, seventeen Buddy Walks took place around the country. Today, there are over two hundred and fifty Buddy Walks around the world. You can find people with Down syndrome and their friends and families organizing these fundraising and awareness walks in Japan, New Zealand, Trinidad, Tobago, Bahamas, and Istanbul! Globally, over 330,000 people gather to walk and celebrate with music and refreshments, guest speakers, and fun activities for kids.

Each year, NDSS announces one or two Grand Marshals to lead the year's New York City Buddy Walk. In 2023, fifteen-year-old hip-hop dancer Macyn Hope Arpi Avis was named Grand Marshal along with nineteen-year-old advocate and public speaker Malik Jabbaar. Just as kids did in 1995, Malik and Macyn stood under their larger-than-life photos on two jumbotrons in the middle of crowded Times Square. Malik flashed a big smile over a sign he held that read in blue and yellow letters, "Just downright awesome!"

In 2023, photos of five hundred different people around the country with Down syndrome appeared on the jumbotron. Afterward, Buddy Walk participants boarded a bus that took them to Central Park. In that vast park full of trees and flowers and birds and squirrels, they stood and listened to the national anthem. Fourteen-year-old Mia Rodriguez, an actor, singer, and activist with Down syndrome, stood onstage in front of thousands of people and sang the anthem.

Following the opening ceremony, Buddy Walk participants typically run, walk, or use wheelchairs or strollers on a mile-long route. Many people wear blue and yellow T-shirts, the official colors of the Down syndrome community. They wave to cheering onlookers on the sidelines, some of whom ask about the walk and then register right then and there to be a part of the fun. After the walk, it's time to party! People play carnival games and explore various stations and booths. Often, entertainers with Down syndrome are invited to put on a show. (For example, at the 2023 New York event, TikTok star Arik Ancelin, a twenty-one-year-old rapper with Down syndrome, entertained the crowd.)

Anyone can participate in a Buddy Walk. You can walk or cheer from the sidelines, run a booth, distribute snacks, or offer to play music. Visit your local Down syndrome advocacy group's webpage to ask about their next walk. Maybe your school, sports team, or scouting club would like to be a walking team or even start a Buddy Walk? You can reach out to the NDSS to find out more information.

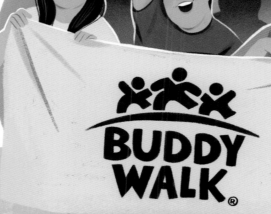

QUICK FACTS ABOUT DOWN SYNDROME

Most of us have forty-six chromosomes in our body—twenty-three pairs. People with Down syndrome have an extra copy of their twenty-first chromosome, which is why it is a genetic condition.

Babies born with Down syndrome have a different number of *chromosomes* than others.

✱ Chromosomes contain our *genes*.

✱ Genes contain our *traits,* or characteristics passed down to us from our parents.

People with Down syndrome are born all over the world.

✱ Approximately six thousand babies are born with Down syndrome *each year in the U.S.*

A British doctor named John Langdon Down first described the genetic condition in 1862.

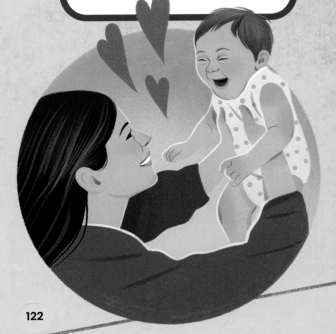

In 2020, archaeologists found the skeleton of a boy with Down syndrome who died between four thousand and six thousand years ago.

Some people with Down syndrome are born with a heart defect or narrow ear canals; both of these conditions often require infant surgery.

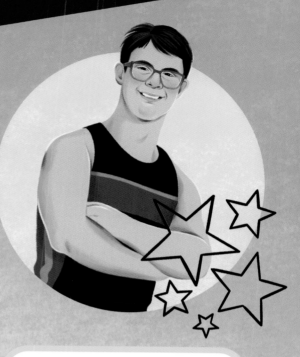

People with Down syndrome share some of the same physical characteristics. These include:

* Small hands and feet
* Small ears
* A short neck
* Almond-shaped eyes that tilt up
* A flattened nose bridge
* A straight line across the palm of each hand.

It may take kids with Down syndrome longer than their peers to walk, talk, read, and write. They benefit from extra help at home and school.

Babies with Down syndrome have low muscle tone, which can be improved with a healthy diet and physical therapy as they grow.

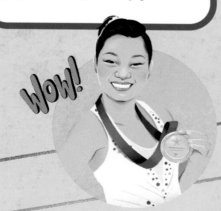

WOW!

People with Down syndrome can play sports, join clubs, sing, act, and do physical activities like dancing, riding bikes, and swimming...
In short, they can do all the things their peers without Down syndrome *can do!*

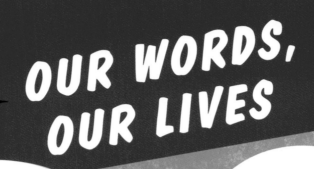

OUR WORDS, OUR LIVES

"Having Down syndrome was not a big deal to me. I'm a businesswoman. I'm the boss, a manager, and the CEO—and a chef."

Allison Fogarty, chef at Doggy Delights by Allison

"Never let anyone's low expectations limit your success."

Abigail Adams, triathlete and activist

"Don't limit us. Don't limit me."

Jamie Brewer, actor

"I have one chromosome more than you. So what?"

Karen Gaffney, swimmer and activist

"Down syndrome never holds me back. I love inspiring people."

John Cronin, cofounder of John's Crazy Socks

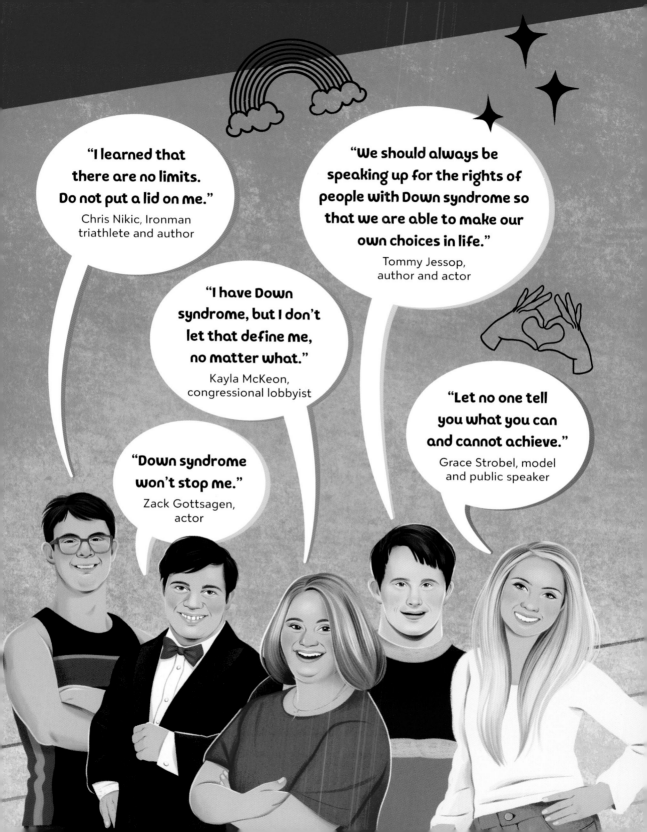

DOWN SYNDROME DISCOVERIES AND DEVELOPMENTS

1838/1839
French doctors describe some characteristics of Down syndrome in their writing.

1866
British doctor John Langdon Down provides a full description of the characteristics of Down syndrome. The condition is named after him.

1929
The life expectancy of someone with Down syndrome is nine years old.

1946
Author Benjamin Spock says parents should put infants born with Down syndrome into institutions instead of raising them at home.

1959
French physician Jérôme Lejeune finds that Down syndrome is caused by an extra twenty-first chromosome.

1968
Eunice Kennedy Shriver and her staff launch the first Special Olympics games.

1970
The life expectancy of someone with Down syndrome is twenty-five years old.

1974
Scientists create the first mouse model with Down syndrome for research. Over the next five decades, they experiment with mice, hoping to understand and improve the lives of people with Down syndrome.

1973
The National Down Syndrome Congress is formed to offer support and information about the genetic condition.

1979

Researchers at the University of Washington show that kids with Down syndrome who are raised at home have a much higher IQ than those raised in institutions.

1979

Barton and Betsy Goodwin establish the National Down Syndrome Society to educate the public and support people with the condition and their families.

1987

Scientists find a gene associated with Alzheimer's disease on chromosome 21, confirming that people with Down syndrome are susceptible to the disease in later life.

1992

Lutheran General Hospital launches the Adult Down Syndrome Center, the first clinic for adults with Down syndrome.

1997

Patricia C. Winders publishes a book called *Gross Motor Skills for Children with Down Syndrome*. The therapies in the book help prevent hip and knee issues in kids with the condition, allowing them to play sports and participate in other physical activities.

2006

The life expectancy of a person with Down syndrome is sixty years.

2020

Geneticists study the DNA preserved in the skeleton of a boy buried between four thousand and six thousand years ago and discover the extra chromosome that causes Down syndrome. It's the oldest documented case of someone with the condition.

2022

Actor and advocate John Franklin Stephens raises money for Alzheimer's disease research on behalf of the Global Down Syndrome Foundation. He also participates in research studies conducted by the Human Trisome Project to help scientists measure brain changes in people with the condition.

THE DISABILITY MOVEMENT IN THE U.S.

1930
Sixty thousand people with intellectual or developmental disabilities (IDD) live in large U.S. institutions.

1950
140,000 people with IDD live in U.S. institutions.

1950s
Parents of people with IDD start a support group called The ARC of the United States.

1960
President John F. Kennedy, whose sister Rosemary has IDD, launches a panel focused on putting people with IDD into small community-based group homes rather than in large institutions.

1958
President Dwight D. Eisenhower passes federal legislation to fund university programs designed to help teachers learn to work with students who have IDD.

1968
The first Special Olympics Games, founded by Eunice Kennedy Shriver, are held in Chicago.

1971
A landmark court case in Pennsylvania supports the rights of all kids with IDD to receive education in public schools.

1972
Journalist Geraldo Rivera exposes the abusive conditions endured by people with IDD at a New York–based institution called Willowbrook State School.

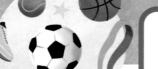

1975
President Gerald Ford passes a law mandating that all public schools provide a complete education to children with disabilities.

1976
The Disability Rights Center is established in Washington, DC.

1981
A feature film titled *Bill* tells the story of Bill Sackter, a man with IDD who ran Wild Bill's Coffee Shop on the University of Iowa campus. The movie shows viewers that people with IDD are capable of holding meaningful jobs and making significant contributions to their communities.

1987
The Willowbrook State School finally closes.

1989
Life Goes On becomes the first network TV series to feature a character with Down syndrome—Corky—played by actor Chris Burke.

1990
The Americans with Disabilities Act (ADA) protects the civil rights of all people with disabilities.

1995
The National Down Syndrome Society launches the first Buddy Walk in Central Park, NY.

1993
The mother of Zack Gottsagen, who would later star in *The Peanut Butter Falcon*, files a lawsuit through the ADA. As a result, all Little League coaches and assistant coaches are required to receive mandatory training in how to include children with disabilities on their teams.

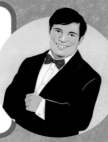

2004
Legislation mandates that students with IDD in public schools must be involved, at least part of the day, in general classrooms.

2010
President Barack Obama mandates the removal of the words *mental retardation* and *mentally retarded* from federal legislation.

2021
U.S. senators introduce the Charlotte Woodward Organ Transplant Discrimination Prevention Act to prevent healthcare providers from discriminating against people with disabilities who require an organ transplant. It's named for Woodward, a person with IDD who received a heart transplant in 2012.

2012
The United Nations recognizes World Down Syndrome Day, an event to be observed on March 21 each year. People with Down syndrome and their families and friends celebrate the day with community service and parties.

2023
The National Down Syndrome Society brings three hundred and fifty activists with IDD to DC's Capitol Hill for the annual Down Syndrome Advocacy Conference.

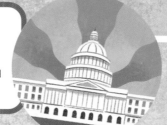

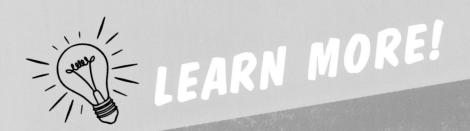

LEARN MORE!

ARE YOU INTRIGUED by the people you've read about in this book? The resources below will deepen your understanding of Down syndrome. You'll learn that people with this genetic condition are excellent students, family members, and friends. And you'll find that including peers with Down syndrome in your friendship circles makes everyone's life better!

MAGAZINES

Down Syndrome World
3.21

FILM & TV

The Peanut Butter Falcon
Champions
Born This Way
Amber and Me

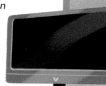

PODCASTS

Special Chronicles
(specialchronicles.com/begin)
Brains On!
"What is Down Syndrome?" (brain-son.org, October 4, 2017)
Stuff You Should Know
"How Down Syndrome Works"
(December 1, 2022)

ORGANIZATIONS

National Down Syndrome Society
(ndss.org)
Global Down Syndrome Society
(globaldownsyndrome.org)
Special Olympics
(specialolympics.org)
National Down Syndrome Congress
(ndsccenter.org)
Gigi's Playhouse
(gigisplayhouse.org)

BOOKS

Nonfiction

Far from the Tree: How Children and Their Parents Learn to Accept One Another...Our Differences Unite Us by Laurie Calkhoven and Andrew Solomon

More Alike Than Different: My Life with Down Syndrome by David and Kathleen Egan

A Life Worth Living: Acting, Activism, and Everything Else by Tommy Jessop

Count Us In: Growing Up with Down Syndrome by Jason Kingsley and Michael Levitz

1% Better: Reaching My Full Potential and How You Can Too by Chris Nikic, Nik Nikic, and Don Yeager

I Am Connor by Conner Rodriguez, Fred Rodriguez, and Marian Tinnelly

You Are Enough: A Book about Inclusion by Sofia Sanchez and Margaret O'Hair

You Are Loved: A Book about Families by Sofia Sanchez and Margaret O'Hair

Fiction

Born to Sparkle: A Story about Achieving Your Dreams by Megan Bomgaars

Marcus Vega Doesn't Speak Spanish by Pablo Cartaya

A Storm of Strawberries by Jo Cotterill

Rosie Loves Jack by Mel Darbon

Collette in Kindergarten by Collette Divitto

Avenging the Owl by Melissa Hart

Daisy Woodworm Changes the World by Melissa Hart

Sing Fox to Me by Sarah Kanake

Pack of Dorks by Beth Vrabel

Hannah's Down Syndrome Superpowers by Lori Leigh Yarborough

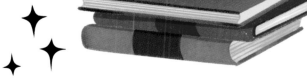

INDEX

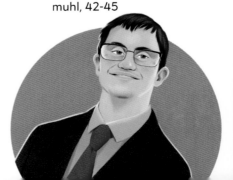

ACKNOWLEDGMENTS

This book has been decades in the making. Long ago, I taught my brother, Mark, how to read and write when people believed that those with Down syndrome couldn't learn these skills. I'm grateful to our mother for raising her kids with equal expectations and equal love, and I'm full of admiration for Mark and our daily conversations about Special Olympics, bowling, and Marvel movies.

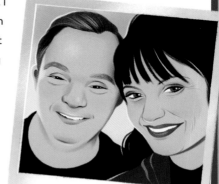

Thank you to my lovely longtime agent, Jennifer Unter, who shared my vision for this book as soon as I proposed it, and to my editor Anna Sargeant, who approached the project with incredible passion for the subject matter and my vision. Thanks to phenomenal illustrator María Diaz Perera, who brought the subjects of this book to life with skill and sensitivity.

Thanks also to Shara Zaval, Maryn Arreguín, and Jessica Nordskog for believing in this book and helping to get it out into the world. Thanks to my friends and colleagues Amy Silverman and George Estreich, whose writing about their children with Down syndrome has long been an inspiration for my work.

Thanks to my daughter, Maia, for listening to the stories that went into this book before I wrote them down. Special thanks to my husband, Jonathan, who took me camping and kayaking to clear my head and who championed this book while applauding my brother's spot-on impressions of the Three Stooges.

I'm especially grateful for the time and energy each person in this book gave me. They and their parents and siblings have been incredibly generous in sharing their stories; because of them, working on this project has been an absolute delight.

ABOUT THE AUTHOR

Melissa Hart grew up near Los Angeles with a younger brother who has Down syndrome. They loved to spend time together, singing and playing guitar, watching movies, and going on nature walks. Melissa worked as a special education teacher for ten years, helping children and adults to achieve their full potential in the classroom and workplace. She lives in Oregon with her husband and daughter, plus a whole lot of cats and chickens and one very patient rescue terrier. Melissa loves to run and hike, bicycle, kayak, and cross-country ski. Find out more about her at www.melissahart.com.

ABOUT THE ILLUSTRATOR

María Perera was born in Gijón, a small town in the north of Spain. At a very young age, she found out that there were few things in life she enjoyed as much as listening to the Beatles and drawing. When she grew up, she graduated from art history at the University of Oviedo, and soon after, she studied graphic design at the Art School of Avilés. Nowadays she still listens to the Beatles and feels fortunate to be able to do what she loves the most for a living: illustration!

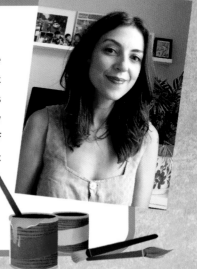